Assistance Robotics and Biosensors 2019

Assistance Robotics and Biosensors 2019

Special Issue Editors
Andrés Úbeda
Fernando Torres Medina
Santiago Puente

MDPI • Basel • Beijing • Wuhan • Barcelona • Belgrade • Manchester • Tokyo • Cluj • Tianjin

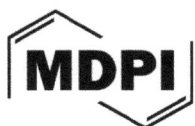

Special Issue Editors

Andrés Úbeda
Human Robotics Group,
University of Alicante
Spain

Fernando Torres Medina
Automatics, Robotics and
Computer Vision Group,
University of Alicante
Spain

Santiago Puente
Automatics, Robotics and
Computer Vision Group,
University of Alicante
Spain

Editorial Office
MDPI
St. Alban-Anlage 66
4052 Basel, Switzerland

This is a reprint of articles from the Special Issue published online in the open access journal *Sensors* (ISSN 1424-8220) (available at: https://www.mdpi.com/journal/sensors/special_issues/arb_2019).

For citation purposes, cite each article independently as indicated on the article page online and as indicated below:

LastName, A.A.; LastName, B.B.; LastName, C.C. Article Title. *Journal Name* **Year**, *Article Number*, Page Range.

ISBN 978-3-03936-417-6 (Hbk)
ISBN 978-3-03936-418-3 (PDF)

© 2020 by the authors. Articles in this book are Open Access and distributed under the Creative Commons Attribution (CC BY) license, which allows users to download, copy and build upon published articles, as long as the author and publisher are properly credited, which ensures maximum dissemination and a wider impact of our publications.

The book as a whole is distributed by MDPI under the terms and conditions of the Creative Commons license CC BY-NC-ND.

Contents

About the Special Issue Editors vii

Andrés Úbeda, Fernando Torres and Santiago T. Puente
Assistance Robotics and Biosensors 2019
Reprinted from: *Sensors* **2020**, *20*, 1335, doi:10.3390/s20051335 1

Nadia Nasri, Sergio Orts-Escolano, Francisco Gomez-Donoso and Miguel Cazorla
Inferring Static Hand Poses from a Low-Cost Non-Intrusive sEMG Sensor
Reprinted from: *Sensors* **2019**, *19*, 371, doi:10.3390/s19020371 5

Dennis Yeung, Dario Farina and Ivan Vujaklija
Directional Forgetting for Stable Co-Adaptation in Myoelectric Control
Reprinted from: *Sensors* **2019**, *19*, 2203, doi:10.3390/s19092203 19

Andrea Gonzalez-Rodriguez, Jose L. Ramon, Vicente Morell, Gabriel J. Garcia, Jorge Pomares, Carlos A. Jara and Andres Ubeda
Evaluation of Optimal Vibrotactile Feedback for Force-Controlled Upper Limb Myoelectric Prostheses
Reprinted from: *Sensors* **2019**, *19*, 5209, doi:10.3390/s19235209 33

Eloy Urendes, Guillermo Asín-Prieto, Ramón Ceres, Rodrigo Garcia-Carmona, Rafael Raya and Jose L. Pons
HYBRID: Ambulatory Robotic Gait Trainer with Movement Induction and Partial Weight Support
Reprinted from: *Sensors* **2019**, *19*, 4773, doi:10.3390/s19214773 43

Sergio D. Sierra M., Mario Garzón, Marcela Múnera and Carlos A. Cifuentes
Human–Robot–Environment Interaction Interface for Smart Walker Assisted Gait: AGoRA Walker
Reprinted from: *Sensors* **2019**, *19*, 2897, doi:10.3390/s19132897 65

Francisco J. Badesa, Jorge A. Diez, Jose Maria Catalan, Emilio Trigili, Francesca Cordella, Marius Nann, Simona Crea, Surjo R. Soekadar, Loredana Zollo, Nicola Vitiello and Nicolas Garcia-Aracil
Physiological Responses During Hybrid BNCI Control of an Upper-Limb Exoskeleton
Reprinted from: *Sensors* **2019**, *19*, 4931, doi:10.3390/s19224931 95

María Elvira, Eduardo Iáñez, Vicente Quiles, Mario Ortiz and José M. Azorín
Pseudo-Online BMI Based on EEG to Detect the Appearance of Sudden Obstacles during Walking
Reprinted from: *Sensors* **2019**, *19*, 5444, doi:10.3390/s19245444 111

Nina Rudigkeit and Marion Gebhard
AMiCUS—A Head Motion-Based Interface for Control of an Assistive Robot
Reprinted from: *Sensors* **2019**, *19*, 2836, doi:10.3390/s19122836 129

About the Special Issue Editors

Andrés Úbeda, PhD in Bioengineering. Andrés Úbeda is an assistant professor in the Department of Physics, System Engineering, and Signal Theory at the University of Alicante (Spain) and a member of the research group Human Robotics. He holds a MSc in Industrial Engineering from the University Miguel Hernández (Spain) (2009), and a PhD in Bioengineering from the same university (2014). He has been a visiting researcher at the Defitech Chair in Non-Invasive Brain–Machine Interfaces (CNBI) at EPFL (École Polytechnique Fédérale de Lausanne, Switzerland) (May–July 2013), at the Institute of Neurorehabilitation Systems (Universitätsmedizin Göttingen, Germany) (Sep 2015–Sep 2016), and the Department of Bioengineering (Imperial College London, UK). He is currently a member of IEEE and the International Society of Electrophysiology and Kinesiology (ISEK). Since January 2020, he has been the IEEE Student Branch Counselor at the University of Alicante. With more than 25 JCR publications, his main research is focused on studying the neuromuscular mechanisms of motor control and coordination, by assessing the descending motor pathways during movement execution. His other research topics are centered on the analysis of cortical information in the decoding of motor intentions, and their use in motor neuro-rehabilitation procedures, human–machine interaction, and assistive technologies in the field of neuro-robotics, particularly focused on myoelectric and brain-controlled devices.

Fernando Torres, PhD Industrial Engineering. Fernando Torres was born in Granada, where he attended primary and high school. He moved to Madrid to undertake a degree in Industrial Engineering at the Polytechnic University of Madrid, where he also carried out his PhD thesis. In the last year of his PhD thesis, he became a full-time lecturer and researcher at the University of Alicante, and he has worked there ever since. He is currently a professor at that University. He directs the research group, "Automatics, Robotics, and Artificial Vision", which was founded in 1996 at the University of Alicante. His research focuses on automation and robotics (intelligent robotic manipulation, visual control of robots, robot perception systems, neurorobotics, field robots and advanced automation for industry 4.0, and artificial vision engineering), and e-learning. In these areas, he has contributed to more than fifty publications in JCR (ISI) journals and more than a hundred papers in international congresses. In addition, he is a member of TC 5.1 and TC 9.4 of the IFAC, a Senior Member of the IEEE, and a member of CEA. He has been the deputy director of the EPS, deputy director of the department, and director of the secretariat at the University of Alicante. He was deputy of the field of Electrical, Electronic, and Automatic Engineering (IEL) at the National Agency of Evaluation and Prospective (ANEP) from 2009 to 2011, and, from 2012 to February 2016, he was the coordinator of this IEL area at the National Agency of Evaluation and Prospective (ANEP). During 2018, he was the coordinator of the field of Electrical, Electronic, and Automatic Evaluation of the ANECA. Since July 2018, he has been the coordinator of the field of Electrical, Electronic, and Automatic (IEA) of the Spanish Agency of State Research (AEI). He served as the coordinator of the Degree in Robotic Engineering at the University of Alicante, from its establishment until 2019, which is the first degree of Robotic Engineering in Spain.

Santiago Puente, PhD Applied Computing. Santiago Puente was born in La Coruña. He moved to Alicante, where he attended primary, high school, and undertook a degree in Computer Engineering at the University of Alicante, where he also carried out his PhD thesis. He obtained a grand to perform his PhD thesis. After one year, he became a full-time lecturer and researcher at the University of Alicante, and he has worked there ever since. He is currently a professor at this University. He is a research member of the research group "Automatics, Robotics, and Artificial Vision", founded in 1996 at the University of Alicante. His research focuses on robotics (intelligent robotic manipulation, neurorobotics, myoelectric control, dexterous grasping, marine robots, and automatic disassembly), deep-learning and e-learning. In these fields, he currently has more than twenty publications in JCR (ISI) journals and nearly a hundred papers in congresses. In addition, he is a member of CEA. He has been deputy director of the EPS since 2013. He is the coordinator of the Degree in Robotic Engineering at the University of Alicante, which is the first degree in Robotic Engineering in Spain, from 2019.

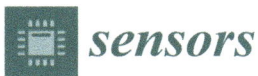

Editorial

Assistance Robotics and Biosensors 2019

Andrés Úbeda [1],*, Fernando Torres [2] and Santiago T. Puente [2]

[1] Human Robotics Group, Department of Physics, System Engineering and Signal Theory, University of Alicante, 03690 Alicante, Spain
[2] AUROVA Group, Department of Physics, System Engineering and Signal Theory, University of Alicante, 03690 Alicante, Spain; fernando.torres@ua.es (F.T.); santiago.puente@ua.es (S.T.P.)
* Correspondence: andres.ubeda@ua.es

Received: 21 February 2020; Accepted: 25 February 2020; Published: 29 February 2020

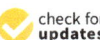

Abstract: This Special Issue is focused on breakthrough developments in the field of assistive and rehabilitation robotics. The selected contributions include current scientific progress from biomedical signal processing and cover applications to myoelectric prostheses, lower-limb and upper-limb exoskeletons and assistive robotics.

Keywords: electromyographic (EMG) sensors; electroencephalographic (EEG) sensors; assistance robotics applications; robotic exoskeletons; robotic prostheses; advanced biomedical signal processing

1. Introduction

In recent years, the use of robotics to help motor-disabled people has experienced a significant growth, mostly based on the development and improvement of biosensor technology and the increasing interest in solving accessibility and rehabilitation limitations in a more natural and effective way. For this purpose, biomedical signal processing has been combined with robotic technology, such as exoskeletons or assistive robotic arms or hands. However, efforts are still needed to make these technologies affordable and useful for end users, as current biomedical devices are still mostly present in rehabilitation centers, hospitals and research facilities. This Special Issue covers several of the recent advances in robotic devices applied to motor rehabilitation and assistance.

2. Contributions

The Special Issue has collected eight outstanding papers covering different aspects of assistance robotics and biosensors. The selected contributions cover several main topics related to assistance robotics, from the control of myoelectric prostheses to the rehabilitation and assistance of the lower and upper limbs. What follows is a brief summary of the scope and main contributions of each of these papers, provided as a teaser for the interested reader.

Upper-limb transradial amputation is cause of severe disability, and a key technology to solve this issue is the use of prosthetic devices for motor substitution. A particular way of controlling these devices is through electromyographic (EMG) signals. In [1], a low-cost non-intrusive myoelectric control is proposed by applying gated recurrent neural networks to data collected from a MYO Armband. This study achieves a 77.85% accuracy when classifying six different hand movements with a generalized classification model.

Other issues that affect classification accuracy are evaluated in [2,3]. An adaptive classification model based on directional forgetting is proposed in [2]. This novel algorithm addresses signal instability issues through a calibration of the model in time, showing good results in a small number of volunteers. Another key factor in myoelectric control is the introduction of an adequate force feedback for the prosthesis. In [3], vibrotactile actuators are used to assess the optimal force feedback patterns delivered to the user. This study reflects that changes in amplitude and frequency level do not show significant differences in the discrimination of vibration patterns. On the other hand, a reduced number of vibration levels increases detection accuracy. Authors propose this study as a starting point for the future optimization of training protocols and for the evaluation of the location and number of vibrotactile actuators.

The rehabilitation of the lower limb has been addressed using a variety of devices, from exoskeletons to walkers. Lower-limb exoskeletons are mainly used in gait rehabilitation. HYBRID is an ambulatory robotic gait trainer with movement induction and partial weight support [4]. This device combines a conventional lower-limb exoskeleton, H1, with an active partial body weight support system (PBWS) to improve locomotive capabilities and minimize muscular effort. This device has proven to be feasible in future clinical applications. Another approach to walking assistance is AGORA [5]. It is a robotic walker (smart walker) that includes several system modules: navigation, human detection, safety, user interaction and social interaction. All these modules are ruled by shared control strategies that command the correct ambulation of the patient.

In [6], the authors propose a method to detect the appearance of sudden obstacles from electroencephalographic (EEG) signals. This method could be applied in the supervision of gait rehabilitation using exoskeletons. The EEG data collected from healthy subjects was processed and classified using linear discriminant analysis, showing an average detection rate of obstacle appearance of about 63.9%, with a false positive rate of 2.6 obstacles per minute. These results were a promising improvement compared to previous studies.

In upper-limb rehabilitation, the physiological interaction of the patient with the robotic device is critical. In [7], two different physiological control methods based on EEG and electrooculography (EOG) are evaluated, while measuring stress levels from skin conductance level (SCL) and heart rate variability (HRV). This study shows that EEG control is associated with a higher level of stress and mental workload when compared to EOG control. An alternative human-robot interaction method is shown in [8]. AMICUS is a head motion-based interface for the control of an assistive robot. In this study, the device is tested by both healthy and tetraplegic participants to perform pick-and-place tasks. The results show that the head motion control is smooth and precise, deriving a high user acceptance.

Acknowledgments: The authors of the submissions have expressed their appreciation of the work of the anonymous reviewers and the *Sensors* editorial team for their cooperation, suggestions and advice. Likewise, the special editors of this Special Issue thank the staff of *Sensors* for the trust shown and the good work that has been done.

Conflicts of Interest: The authors declare no conflict of interest.

References

1. Nasri, N.; Orts-Escolano, S.; Gomez-Donoso, F.; Cazorla, M. Inferring Static Hand Poses from a Low-Cost Non-Intrusive sEMG Sensor. *Sensors* **2019**, *19*, 371. [CrossRef] [PubMed]
2. Yeung, D.; Farina, D.; Vujaklija, I. Directional Forgetting for Stable Co-Adaptation in Myoelectric Control. *Sensors* **2019**, *19*, 2203. [CrossRef] [PubMed]
3. Gonzalez-Rodriguez, A.; Ramon, J.; Morell, V.; Garcia, G.; Pomares, J.; Jara, C.; Ubeda, A. Evaluation of Optimal Vibrotactile Feedback for Force-Controlled Upper Limb Myoelectric Prostheses. *Sensors* **2019**, *19*, 5209. [CrossRef] [PubMed]
4. Urendes, E.; Asín-Prieto, G.; Ceres, R.; García-Carmona, R.; Raya, R.; L. Pons, J. HYBRID: Ambulatory Robotic Gait Trainer with Movement Induction and Partial Weight Support. *Sensors* **2019**, *19*, 4773. [CrossRef] [PubMed]
5. Sierra, M.S.; Garzón, M.; Múnera, M.; Cifuentes, C. Human–Robot–Environment Interaction Interface for Smart Walker Assisted Gait: AGoRA Walker. *Sensors* **2019**, *19*, 2897. [CrossRef] [PubMed]
6. Badesa, F.; Diez, J.; Catalan, J.; Trigili, E.; Cordella, F.; Nann, M.; Crea, S.; Soekadar, S.; Zollo, L.; Vitiello, N.; et al. Physiological Responses During Hybrid BNCI Control of an Upper-Limb Exoskeleton. *Sensors* **2019**, *19*, 4931. [CrossRef] [PubMed]

7. Elvira, M.; Iáñez, E.; Quiles, V.; Ortiz, M.; Azorín, J. Pseudo-Online BMI Based on EEG to Detect the Appearance of Sudden Obstacles during Walking. *Sensors* **2019**, *19*, 5444. [CrossRef] [PubMed]
8. Rudigkeit, N.; Gebhard, M. AMiCUS—A Head Motion-Based Interface for Control of an Assistive Robot. *Sensors* **2019**, *19*, 2836. [CrossRef] [PubMed]

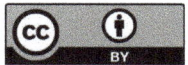 © 2020 by the authors. Licensee MDPI, Basel, Switzerland. This article is an open access article distributed under the terms and conditions of the Creative Commons Attribution (CC BY) license (http://creativecommons.org/licenses/by/4.0/).

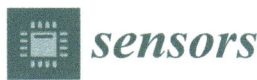

Article

Inferring Static Hand Poses from a Low-Cost Non-Intrusive sEMG Sensor

Nadia Nasri *, Sergio Orts-Escolano, Francisco Gomez-Donoso and Miguel Cazorla

University Institute for Computer Research, University of Alicante, P.O. Box 99, 03080 Alicante, Spain; sorts@ua.es (S.O.-E.); fgomez@dccia.ua.es (F.G.-D.); miguel.cazorla@ua.es (M.C.)
* Correspondence: nnasri@dccia.ua.es

Received: 28 November 2018; Accepted: 15 January 2019; Published: 17 January 2019

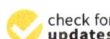

Abstract: Every year, a significant number of people lose a body part in an accident, through sickness or in high-risk manual jobs. Several studies and research works have tried to reduce the constraints and risks in their lives through the use of technology. This work proposes a learning-based approach that performs gesture recognition using a surface electromyography-based device, the Myo Armband released by Thalmic Labs, which is a commercial device and has eight non-intrusive low-cost sensors. With 35 able-bodied subjects, and using the Myo Armband device, which is able to record data at about 200 MHz, we collected a dataset that includes six dissimilar hand gestures. We used a gated recurrent unit network to train a system that, as input, takes raw signals extracted from the surface electromyography sensors. The proposed approach obtained a 99.90% training accuracy and 99.75% validation accuracy. We also evaluated the proposed system on a test set (new subjects) obtaining an accuracy of 77.85%. In addition, we showed the test prediction results for each gesture separately and analyzed which gestures for the Myo armband with our suggested network can be difficult to distinguish accurately. Moreover, we studied for first time the gated recurrent unit network capability in gesture recognition approaches. Finally, we integrated our method in a system that is able to classify live hand gestures.

Keywords: surface electromyography sensor; dataset; gated recurrent units; gesture recognition

1. Introduction

The importance of technology and science in improving the quality of human health and facilitating human life has been amply demonstrated [1,2]. According to information from the LN-4 project (https://ln-4.org/), the amputee population can be estimated at 1.5 per 1000 persons and 30% of these are arm amputees [3]. In this case, using an upper-limb prosthesis is a popular solution. The main objective of this work is a system for amputees that can also be used as a robot remote control.

Most of the deployed cosmetic prosthetics resemble an arm or hand simply to offset the space left by the amputated limb. Fortunately, with constantly improving technology, efforts are focused on creating several variants of robotic arms and hands that could replace the lost limb with similar characteristics to a real hand in both appearance and movements. The prostheses available need complicated, cumbersome, expensive equipment, reducing demand.

However, the methods for controlling robotic prosthetics are a topic of interest in the literature. In addition, most of the control methods require surgery to be implanted for good prosthetic performance, and are intended to be permanent. However, technology advances, modifying and upgrading these mechanisms may be problematic, involving discomfort and significant extra costs. Amputees' health may be endangered and the upgrade capabilities may be technically and economically limited.

There also exist control methods which are non-intrusive and benefit from surface electromyography (sEMG). A surface EMG is a useful non-intrusive technique for recording the electrical activity produced by muscles through surface sensors placed on parts of the body while muscles in that area are active. This technology is currently emerging as a substitute for the above-mentioned intrusive methods to control prosthetic limbs, with a focus on safety precautions against unknown consequences [4–6].

The most recent methods for controlling prosthetics leverage Machine Learning techniques. These classifiers receive labeled data from EMG sensors to learn and recognize the high level features of each pose. Subsequently, they take the output of the EMG sensors in real time shortly after the hand pose, and infer the signals and the features of the pose the user is trying to perform. The pose configuration is then sent to the motors placed in the prosthetic to move and replicate the intended pose.

An issue considered in this research is, the need of a large number of custom EMG sensors in some successful previous studies, and, therefore, their high cost [7,8]. This creates problems for users to access these methods, hence, in the present work, we attempted to create the maximum benefit at the minimum cost. Our proposed framework utilizes the Myo Gesture Control Armband, which is made of low-cost non-intrusive sEMG sensors (existing consumer product released by Thalmic Labs). In addition, this paper aims to expand the research to create a new dataset for six static hand gestures and use Gated Recurrent Unit (GRU) architecture for gesture recognition, which is new approach for this type of architecture.

Human–Robot Interaction (HRI) has been a noteworthy topic of academic research since the 20th century [9]. HRI research spans a wide range of fields dedicated to understanding, designing, and evaluating robotic systems and their services to humanity. There are several methods of human–robot interaction, each of them with their own benefits and deficiencies [10,11].

The main contributions of this paper are:

- The creation of a public dataset containing 35 subjects with six dissimilar hand gestures.
- A method for discrete hand pose classification with sEMG signals. The proposed method is based on deep learning and it obtains a high recognition accuracy.

The method presented in this paper can be used as a teleoperation method that an operator can remote and control a robot meticulously through six static hand gestures with any degree of freedom (DOF) in shoulder joint and elbow (shoulder joint includes three DOF and elbow includes two DOF). Teleoperation methods are useful in several fields, especially in some working environments that are dangerous and not suitable for operators. Several teleoperation methods were proposed [12,13] and there are some works with use of the Myo armband for the purpose of controlling robots with different methods [14–16].

The rest of the paper is organized as follows: Section 2 reviews the state of the art related to existing hand pose datasets, recorded using EMG and sEMG sensors. Moreover, we review existing learning-based approaches/systems that perform hand gesture and pose estimation using sEMG sensors. Next, in Section 3, the details of the capture device and sensor types that we used for composing the dataset are described and relevant details of the process of acquiring datasets are explained. Section 4 describes the system and architecture of the neural network used to train the hand gestures recognition dataset to be used for other hand poses to estimate the success of the system based on the proposals. Section 5 shows the obtained results and describes the experimental process. Section 6 presents the main conclusions of the present work and suggests some objectives for future works.

2. Background and Related Work

Hand gesture recognition via surface (sEMG) sensors placed on the arm has been a subject of considerable research with different features for applications and prosthetics. Quality of life for amputees is highly deficient in comparison to pre amputation (and losing their limb) but can be ameliorated with real-time control systems based on hand movements [17,18].

Nowadays, high-density surface electromyography (HD-sEMG) is of great importance in the medical community [19,20], and has also been used to recognize hand gestures and control muscle–computer interfaces (MCIs) [21–23]. A large number of electrodes are essential [24], although other methods exist which improve recognition accuracies using multi-channel sEMG and HD- sEMG electrodes [25,26].

There are published datasets (See Figure 1) from several studies with a similar aim such as NinaPro (Non Invasive Adaptive Hand Prosthetics) [27], CapgMyo [28] and csl-hdemg [24]. In CapMyo and csl-hdemg, datasets were recorded by a large number of HD-sEMG with a high sampling rate using dense arrays of individual electrodes, in order to obtain information from the muscles [28]. Recently, a significant number of methods have been used which depend on HD-sEMG with 2D electrode arrays for gesture recognition approaches [22,23,29]. The capacity of HD-sEMG is currently the subject of research. Bearing in mind the existence of significant differences between sEMG signal and HD-sEMG results [29], we decided to work with sEMG.

DATASET NAME	SUBJECTS	EMG TYPE	NUMBER OF GESTURES
NinaPro(DB1)	27	10 sEMG(Otto Bock) CyberGlove II	52
NinaPro(DB2)	40	12 sEMG(Delsys) CyberGlove II	50
CapgMyo(DB-a)	18	128 HD-sEMG	8
Csl-hdemg	5	192 HD-sEMG	27 (finger gestures)

Figure 1. Public database summary table.

Datasets which are acquired by HD-sEMG signals are not appropriate under our framework in this research and only NinaPro databases contain regular sEMG electrodes in their recording process. The NinaPro database was recorded from a sample of 78 participants (67 able-bodied persons, 11 trans-radial amputated persons, in three different phases) and 52 different gestures. In this project, 10–12 electrodes (Otto Bock 13-E200 (Ontario, ON, Canada), Delsys Trigno (Natick, MA, USA)) were placed on forearms, plus one CyberGlove II with 22 sensors to capture 3D hand poses. Four classification methods were applied on a five-signal feature. Because of the multiplicity of costly sensors and the various signal processing steps applied on raw sEMG data used in this research, we decided to work with raw signals. The NinaPro dataset does not fit the objective of this work [8]. In the continuation of the NinaPro research and development of their benchmark, a public dataset DB5 was recorded using a double Myo armband and a CyberGlove in order to reduce the expenses of the research with qualified results [30].

An investigation which focused on the evaluation between different machine learning methods exerted on EMG signals [31] provided interesting results and many studies highlight the success of deep learning techniques, especially ConvNet, in hand gesture classification [16,25,32]. They also demonstrate that using ConvNet as a feature extractor from sEMG images (or spectrograms) can achieve qualified accuracy [16,28,32] even with semi-supervised data [25].

EMG signals captured by low-cost Myo armband were used in some recent research [16,30] and were shown to be able to record EMG data. In addition, other works have used Myo armband and its default gesture recognition pattern with a machine learning algorithm to control movements of objects. One of the most recent studies conducted using a Myo armband [33] involved combining the sEMG signal with a Virtual Reality (VR) headset output and implementing Support Vector Machine algorithm to be used for classification. The system was developed to control a robot through eye movements and facial gestures. However, the Myo armband default system in real time has a considerable error rate when recognizing the correct hand pose. Moreover, the number of gestures is limited and the armband contains only five hand gestures.

In the present work, we decided to test raw EMG signals as input of the network. Accordingly, we had to opt for a network which can train with signals. Therefore, we perused recurrent neural network characteristics. As there is little information on using sEMG signals and RNN architectures, we reviewed the results from these architectures with speech signals.

Recurrent neural networks (RNN) have recently proven success in various tasks, especially in machine translation [34,35]. The long short-term memory (LSTM) [36] has shown promising results in a number of natural language processing tasks [34,37], and it was followed by the proposed architecture gated recurrent unit (GRU) [38]. Both architectures have performed well in comparison with ConvNet [39] and on raw speech signal data [40]. Consequently, we decided to utilize sEMG raw signals as an input for our GRU-based network.

3. sEMG Dataset Recording and Processing

We studied a number of public datasets, but their sensors did not fit our objective and framework because of the type of sensor and the high number required. Therefore, we decided to create a new dataset for six static hand gestures recorded by Myo armband with the participation of 35 intact individuals.

3.1. EMG Sensor Type Discussion

There are two kinds of EMG electrodes: Intramuscular EMG and Surface EMG. Intramuscular EMG has various kinds of recording electrodes; applying needle electrodes is a common method of this category. However, the difficulty of placing them on the arm and connecting them with the muscles correctly make this an arduous task and generates pain and risks for users.

Surface EMG category comprises gel-based and dry electrodes. To be able to use gel-based sEMG, a preparation process is needed before placing the electrodes. The skin must be cleaned and the user's arm shaved. A conductor gel must then be applied to receive the ideal captured data from electrodes. As the preparation step is lengthy and intricate, this type of sEMG is not an appropriate option to surmount an amputee's requirements for doing daily routines, which makes them less popular as a long use solution. Although applying dry electrodes reduces preparation time, they still present certain limitations and, with higher impedance, are less accurate compared to gel-based ones [41,42]. Due to the easy access and facilities of handling dry sEMG, in this research, we chose the Myo armband, which has eight dry sEMGs.

3.2. Recording Hardware

In recent years, Thalmic Labs(Kitchener, ON, Canada) released a commercial device, the Myo (https://www.myo.com/) armband (the device is available for public unrestricted purchasing), gesture control device composed of a low-consumption ARM Cortex-M4 120 MHZ microprocessor (ArmDeveloper, Cambridge, United Kingdom), 8 dry sEMG and inertial measurement unit (IMU) with a low-sampling rate (200 Hz) (see Figure 2). It provides two types of output data: spatial data and gestural data. The spatial data records the orientation and movements of the user's arm by 9-axis IMU. Gestural data is recorded by 8 sEMG and gives the information on electrical activity produced by skeletal muscles (This research did not focus on spatial data and just uses EMG data). The use of the Myo armband device has been studied in multiple studies using deep learning architectures [30,43–45].

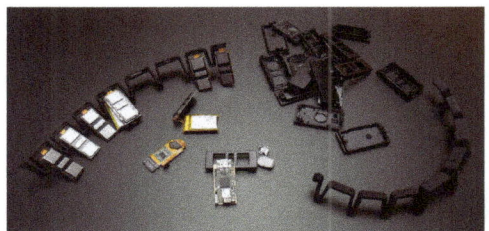

Figure 2. Myo armband tear-down [46].

3.3. Recording and Labeling Data

In this project, 35 healthy and able-bodied subjects cooperated in the recording of data and labeling hand gestures. The dataset was collected from intact persons of different genders, ages and physical conditions (height and weight).

Six dissimilar hand gestures (open hand, closed hand, wrist extension, wrist flexion, tap and victory sign) were chosen to train and test the system (See Figure 3). The Myo armband was placed at the height of the Radio-humeral joint, being calibrated for right forearm and right hand gestures. As Myo seemed stable to the external factors [30], special treatment was not needed to begin the data acquisition. However, many factors can affect the sEMG signals [47,48] and should be considered.

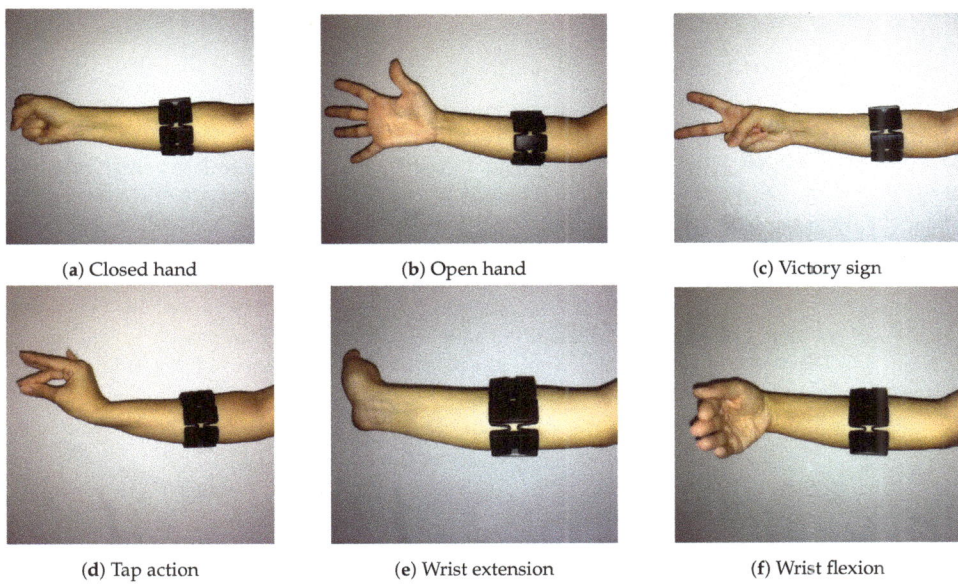

(**a**) Closed hand   (**b**) Open hand   (**c**) Victory sign

(**d**) Tap action   (**e**) Wrist extension   (**f**) Wrist flexion

Figure 3. Hand gestures.

Before the data recording process started, all subjects were given an oral explanation about the experiments and the risks, and were asked to complete an information form. For the sake of completeness and system training, during the data capturing process, one condition was determined. All the subjects were asked to maintain the requested hand gesture, move their arms in various directions for 10 s for each gesture to have more than one Degree Of Freedom (DOF), and avoid complete bending of the forearm at the elbow joint to prevent unwanted effects of brachialis muscle on sEMG signals. Between each gesture recording process, subjects were given a few minutes to rest their arm. Data from Myo was transmitted via Bluetooth at slightly less than 200 Hz in eight channels for each sample (See Figure 4). From the 35 healthy subjects, we acquired approximately 41,000 samples. Twenty-eight subjects were taken for the data training and validation (70% of sample for data training and 30% of sample for data validation), and seven people for test examination whose information was not received by the system during the training process.

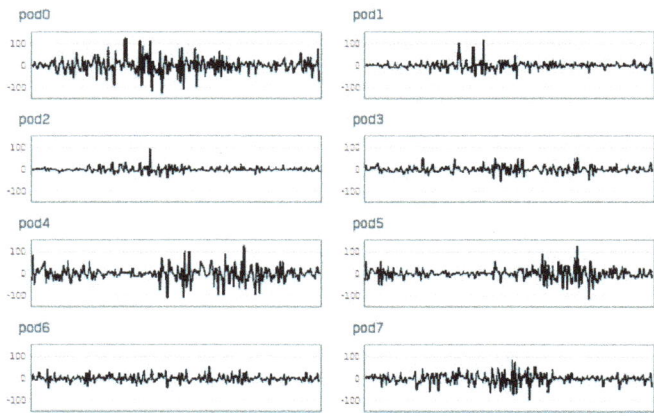

Figure 4. Raw signals (eight) captured with by Myo armband device.

4. System Description

In this work, we used a GRU network to process raw sEMG signals. No pre-processing process on the sEMG signal recorded by Myo was necessary. By default, the recorded signal was normalized in the range of −128 to 127 and other methods of normalization were implemented such as normalizing per channel and normalizing between −1 and 1. Nevertheless, the best accuracy was obtained by using the default output of the armband as it is naturally zero-centered. To achieve a better result, we used the window method. Following this method, multiple recent time steps can be used to make a prediction for the next time step. We tried several quantities for the window method and considered 188 as the look-back per sample which had the best outcome with 20 as offset in each window. The look-back number is dependent on the armband frequency that generates almost 188 samples per second and a second is the estimated time that a subject needs to make the gesture correctly in static hand gestures. Figure 5 corresponds to one of the eight channels that are used.

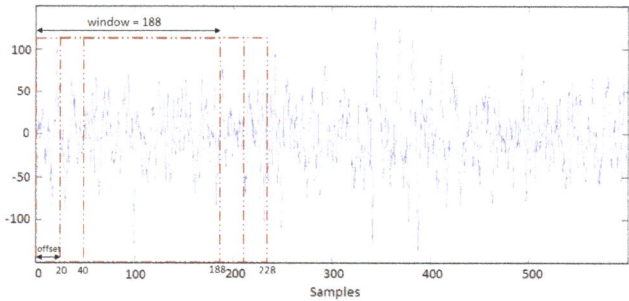

Figure 5. Window method implemented on input data.

Our neural network contains GRU units, dropout and a fully connected layer. The number of GRU units was tested in several training processes regarding the highest accuracy for the data test.

Gated Recurrent Unit Network

In this work, the implemented GRU type is the default one based on [38]; GRU is a variant of LSTM, with fewer parameters and faster processing time. It does not use the memory unit to control the data and its reset gate was applied to the hidden state; it can utilize hidden states freely without observation.

Our proposed classifier follows a recurrent approach. These kinds of methods work with sequences of data to extract temporal features that enable classification cues. Our proposed network features three sequential GRU layers followed by a fully connected layer. Each GRU layer is composed of 150 units with a hyperbolic tangent (tanh) activation function. Each GRU layer is connected to a dropout layer. These layers inhibit random neuron activations with a 0.5 probability. The effect caused by this is twofold: on one hand, the network learns to deal with slightly altered or missing input data. On the other hand, with each iteration, the network is actually training a different architecture as some connections are inhibited. Thus, this layer helps fight overfitting and benefits the generalization capabilities of the final model. Finally, our proposal features a last fully connected (FC) layer with six neurons matching the number of classes of our problem. This final layer is a traditional Multi Layer Perceptron in which neurons have complete linkage to those in the GRU layer's output. The output from GRU carries important features of the sEMG signals and the fully connected layer uses these features to classify the input signal into existing classes based on the training dataset. This layer uses a softmax activation function that helps control the actions of extreme values without omitting them from the dataset. The described architecture is shown in Figure 6.

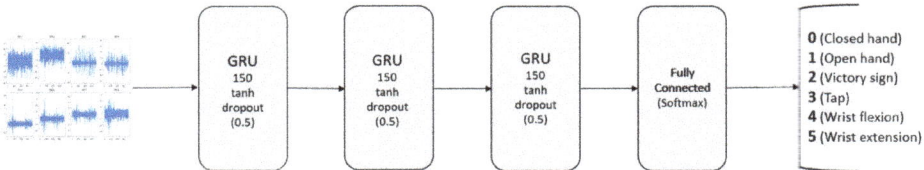

Figure 6. Proposed neural network architecture for hand gesture recognition.

The parameters of the architecture such as number of layers, number of neurons per layer, activation functions, normalization layers and dropout rates were empirically chosen.

Finally, it is worth noting that the input data of the network features a *batch_size* × *time_steps* × *channels* shape. The *batch_size* is the number of samples in one iteration of the training algorithm. In our case, there were 500 samples in each batch. As mentioned, we considered 188 EMG readings per samples, thus *time_steps* corresponds to the second dimension. The *channel* dimension corresponds to the readings of the eight different surface sensors of the Myo armband.

For the loss function, we used the categorical-crossentropy function, which means we received a vector with six dimensions as output, which are all zero except one in the prediction index of gesture classes.

5. Experiments and Results

Initially, in order to choose the most efficient architecture for the neural network, we divided our experiment into two phases. First, we recorded three basic hand gestures with almost 6000 samples from 10 subjects via the armband (closed hand, open hand and victory sign), and examined the output to check the competence of the armband and the GRU network (see Figure 7).

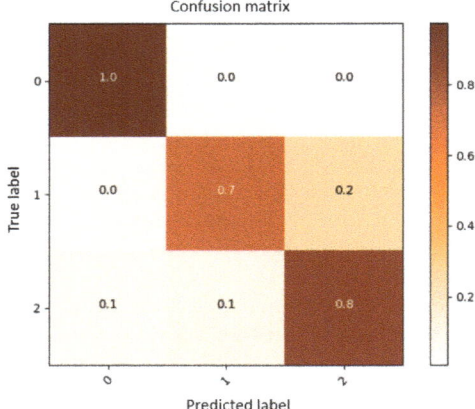

Figure 7. Confusion matrix for three gestures.

Based on the preliminary experiments and in order to expand the dataset, we selected 10 dissimilar hand gestures and trained the network, but the Myo armband and its eight sensors were not sufficient to recognize the difference in all the gestures, with test results being around 40%. According to the evaluation procedure described in previous works [8,30], a Myo armband alone is not enough for more than 6–7 gestures [16] and, for more gestures, it should be combined with at least two separate sEMGs placed on flexor digitorum superficialis and extensor digitorum active spots.

For more realistic results, we divided the dataset into five groups. Subsequently, we implemented the leave-one-out Cross-Validation technique (35 healthy subjects were divided into groups of seven people) and the training process was conducted via GeForce GTX 1080Ti GPU (Santa Clara, CA, USA). As one group was left out per test, the data for the rest of the subjects was shuffled and divided into 70% for training data and 30% for validation data. The system did not see the validation split during the training process and validation data was from the same subjects as training data but with different samples. In all groups, training accuracy was between 99.40–99.97% as can be seen in Figure 8, which means that the system was learning and could distinguish all gestures. Validation accuracy follows training accuracy during the process with an insignificant difference.

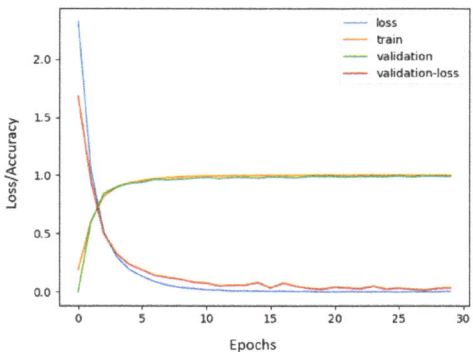

Figure 8. Accuracy and loss graph during the training process.

The Cross-Validation experiment includes the training process repeated five times. Each time, four groups were considered as data training, one group as data testing and all five groups were examined as data tests at different times in order to survey the system more accurately. With respect to the Cross-Validation results, the average test accuracy is estimated to be around 77.85%.

It is worth noting at this point that we adopted an early stopping criteria, so the training processes were halted just before an overfitting event or upon stabilization of losses/accuracies. As a result, all experiments were training for about 300 epochs, which were delayed for about 36 h each in the mentioned GeForce GTX 1080Ti GPU. Finally, the optimizer of choice was Adam with a learning rate starting at 0.0001. As concluded in [49], Adam was the best performer, so we adopted it.

We also implemented a T-distributed Stochastic Neighbor Embedding(T-SNE) algorithm to carry out a dimensionality reduction in 2D for the visualization of our high-dimensional data in Figure 9. In this figure, the training data reduced to two dimensions is plotted. It can be observed that the clusters (different colors indicate different gestures) are separated and, therefore, can be learned by a machine learning method.

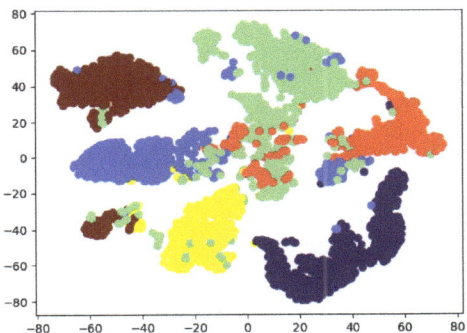

Figure 9. Categorize data by features via T-SNE.

In some groups of features, there are errors, which can be seen in the different colors in Figure 9. This means that the system was unable to predict the gestures correctly.

A more accurate estimation of the error percentage can be seen in the confusion matrix (there is a probability of maximum ±0.05 error in each row or column, due to the rounding of numbers). In accordance with the information educed from the confusion matrix in Figure 10, the supposition that GRU architecture is qualified for the gesture recognition system can be proved. Moreover, the confusion matrices demonstrate that the system for subjects who were trained on different samples (validation data) is reasonably accurate. Then, Figure 10b shows a confusion matrix for the test split. It shows that the proposed system is able to successfully classify proposed hand poses even for new subjects.

As the final experiments in this section to test our proposed architecture for gesture recognition, we implemented a live system. The system receives Myo armband information, passes it through the neural network, loads training weights and infers the hand gestures. We ran the live system for five new subjects and found an average accuracy of 80%. According to the results of the live system, there were inconsistencies only between the Victory-sign gesture and the others; for the remaining gestures, we obtained appropriate results. Regarding the runtime, the system is able to provide a prediction in 42 ms in a GeForce GTX 1050 GPU, which means it performs at about 23 frames per second.

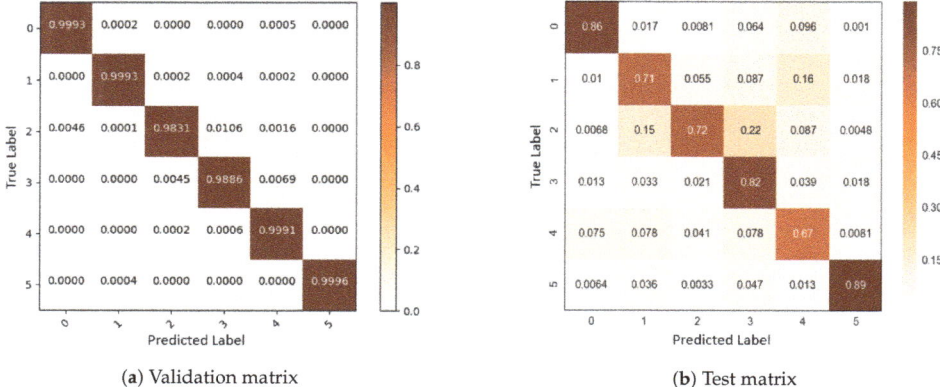

(a) Validation matrix (b) Test matrix

Figure 10. Confusion matrix.

One of the recorded subjects was suffering from Charcot–Marie–Tooth disease (CMT) (https://www.cmtausa.org/understanding-cmt/what-is-cmt/), although he was healthy and had no movement restrictions. We noticed this patient's sEMG signals of the patient were totally dissimilar and inconsistent with those of the other subjects. At different stages, this patient was used as a data test so we could compare his results with the other subjects (See Figure 11). As Johnson et al. indicate, patients with CMT have muscle cramps which could affect sEMG signals [50]. Hence, we decided to replace this patient's data with that of an able-bodied subject in our dataset. This finding suggests there might be probabilities of detecting neuromuscular diseases with this system, which could be studied and developed in future works.

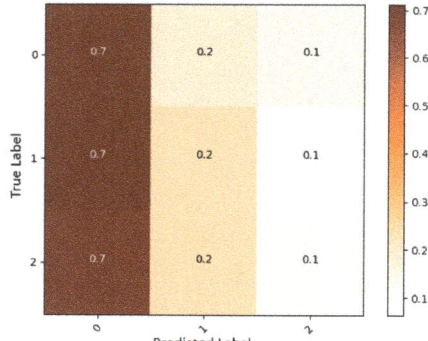

Figure 11. Confusion matrix from a patient with CMT disease.

6. Conclusions

In this paper, we describe a new approach for live gesture classification with GRU architecture trained by sEMG raw signals acquired from the Myo armband. A new dataset containing approximately 41,000 samples for six dissimilar static hand gestures was created. The proposed GRU classifier was evaluated on different validation sets obtaining an accuracy of 77.85%, to be developed and used for classifying a set of hand gestures performed by a human being. We also studied the correct prediction probability for each gesture and their conflict with other gestures. Moreover, we performed live experiments with multiple new users, verifying that the system was able to distinguish approximately 80% of the trained gestures. In addition, according our experiments' results, we showed that the GRU network is accurate enough to be used in gesture recognition systems.

Future works will focus on developing our dataset, augmenting further hand gestures and testing the system to control a prosthetic hand.

Author Contributions: Authors contributed as follows: methodology, N.N. and F.G.-D.; software, F.G.-D.; data acquisition, N.N.; validation, S.O.-E. and M.C.; investigation, N.N.; resources, N.N.; data curation, N.N.; writing–original draft preparation, N.N. and F.G.-D.; writing–review and editing, S.O.-E. and M.C.; visualization, N.N.; supervision, S.O.-E. and M.C.; project administration, M.C.

Funding: This work was supported by the Spanish Government TIN2016-76515R grant, supported with Feder funds. It has also been funded by the University of Alicante project GRE16-19, by the Valencian Government project GV/2018/022, and by a Spanish grant for PhD studies ACIF/2017/243.

Acknowledgments: The authors would like to thank all the subjects for their participation in the data collection experiments. We would also like to thank NVIDIA (Santa Clara, CA, USA) for the generous donation of a Titan Xp and a Quadro P6000.

Conflicts of Interest: The authors declare no conflict of interest.

References

1. Cook, A.M.; Polgar, J.M. *Essentials of Assistive Technologies*; ELSEVIER Mosby: Amsterdam, The Netherlands, 2012.
2. Costa, A.; Martinez-Martin, E.; Cazorla, M.; Julian, V. PHAROS—PHysical Assistant RObot System. *Sensors* **2018**, *18*, 2633. [CrossRef]
3. LeBlanc, M. The LN-4 Prosthetic Hand. In *Give Hope—Give a Hand*; The Ellen Meadows Prosthetic Hand Foundation: San Francisco, CA, USA, 2008.
4. Momen, K.; Krishnan, S.; Chau, T. Real-time classification of forearm electromyographic signals corresponding to user-selected intentional movements for multifunction prosthesis control. *IEEE Trans. Neural Syst. Rehabil. Eng.* **2007**, *15*, 535–542. [CrossRef]
5. Amsuss, S.; Goebel, P.M.; Jiang, N.; Graimann, B.; Paredes, L.; Farina, D. Self-correcting pattern recognition system of surface EMG signals for upper limb prosthesis control. *IEEE Trans. Biomed. Eng.* **2014**, *61*, 1167–1176. [CrossRef]
6. Boostani, R.; Moradi, M.H. Evaluation of the forearm EMG signal features for the control of a prosthetic hand. *Physiol. Meas.* **2003**, *24*, 309. [CrossRef]
7. Gijsberts, A.; Atzori, M.; Castellini, C.; Müller, H.; Caputo, B. Movement Error Rate for Evaluation of Machine Learning Methods for sEMG-Based Hand Movement Classification. *IEEE Trans. Neural Syst. Rehabil. Eng.* **2014**, *22*, 735–744. [CrossRef]
8. Atzori, M.; Gijsberts, A.; Castellini, C.; Caputo, B.; Hager, A.G.M.; Elsig, S.; Giatsidis, G.; Bassetto, F.; Müller, H. Electromyography data for non-invasive naturally-controlled robotic hand prostheses. *Sci. Data* **2014**, *1*, 140053. [CrossRef]
9. Asimov, I. *The Three Laws of Robotics*; Gnome Press: New York, NY, USA, 1941.
10. HRI '11: *Proceedings of the 6th International Conference on Human-robot Interaction, Lausanne, Switzerland, 6–9 March 2011*; ACM: New York, USA, 2011; p. 609114.
11. Scholtz, J. *Human Robot Interactions: Creating Synergistic Cyber Forces*; AAAI Technical Report FS-02-03; Springer: Dordrecht, The Netherlands, 2002.
12. Yang, C.; Chang, S.; Liang, P.; Li, Z.; Su, C.Y. Teleoperated robot writing using EMG signals. In Proceedings of the 2015 IEEE International Conference on Information and Automation, Lijiang, China, 8–10 August 2015; pp. 2264–2269.
13. Reddivari, H.; Yang, C.; Ju, Z.; Liang, P.; Li, Z.; Xu, B. Teleoperation control of Baxter robot using body motion tracking. In Proceedings of the 2014 International Conference on Multisensor Fusion and Information Integration for Intelligent Systems (MFI), Beijing, China, 28–29 September 2014; pp. 1–6. [CrossRef]
14. Xu, Y.; Yang, C.; Liang, P.; Zhao, L.; Li, Z. Development of a hybrid motion capture method using MYO armband with application to teleoperation. In Proceedings of the 2016 IEEE International Conference on Mechatronics and Automation, Harbin, China, 7–10 August 2016; pp. 1179–1184. [CrossRef]
15. Bisi, S.; De Luca, L.; Shrestha, B.; Yang, Z.; Gandhi, V. Development of an EMG-Controlled Mobile Robot. *Robotics* **2018**, *7*, 36. [CrossRef]

16. Allard, U.C.; Nougarou, F.; Fall, C.L.; Giguère, P.; Gosselin, C.; Laviolette, F.; Gosselin, B. A convolutional neural network for robotic arm guidance using semg based frequency-features. In Proceedings of the Intelligent Robots and Systems (IROS), Daejeon, Korea, 9–14 October 2016; pp. 2464–2470.
17. Ahsan, M.D.; Ibrahimy, M.I.; Khalifa, O.O. Advances in Electromyogram Signal Classification to Improve the Quality of Life for the Disabled and Aged People. *J. Comput. Sci.* **2010**, *6*, 706–715. [CrossRef]
18. Brose, S.W.; Weber, D.J.; Salatin, B.A.; Grindle, G.G.; Wang, H.; Vazquez, J.J.; Cooper, R.A. The role of assistive robotics in the lives of persons with disability. *Am. J. Phys. Med. Rehabil.* **2010**, *89*, 509–521. [CrossRef]
19. Blok, J.H.; Van Dijk, J.P.; Drost, G.; Zwarts, M.J.; Stegeman, D.F. A high-density multichannel surface electromyography system for the characterization of single motor units. *Rev. Sci. Instrum.* **2002**, *73*, 1887–1897. [CrossRef]
20. Drost, G.; Stegeman, D.F.; van Engelen, B.G.; Zwarts, M.J. Clinical applications of high-density surface EMG: A systematic review. *J. Electromyogr Kinesiol.* **2006**, *16*, 586–602. [CrossRef]
21. Saponas, T.S.; Tan, D.S.; Morris, D.; Balakrishnan, R. Demonstrating the Feasibility of Using Forearm Electromyography for Muscle-computer Interfaces. In Proceedings of the SIGCHI Conference on Human Factors in Computing Systems, Florence, Italy, 5–10 April 2008; ACM: New York, NY, USA, 2008; pp. 515–524 [CrossRef]
22. Rojas-Martínez, M.; Mañanas, M.A.; Alonso, J.F.; Merletti, R. Identification of isometric contractions based on High Density EMG maps. *J. Electromyogr. Kinesiol.* **2013**, *23*, 33–42. [CrossRef]
23. Zhang, X.; Zhou, P. High-density myoelectric pattern recognition toward improved stroke rehabilitation. *IEEE Trans. Biomed. Eng.* **2012**, *59*, 1649–1657. [CrossRef]
24. Amma, C.; Krings, T.; Böer, J.; Schultz, T. Advancing Muscle-Computer Interfaces with High-Density Electromyography. In Proceedings of the 33rd Annual ACM Conference on Human Factors in Computing Systems, Seoul, Korea, 18–23 April 2015; ACM: New York, NY, USA, 2015; pp. 929–938. [CrossRef]
25. Du, Y.; Wong, Y.; Jin, W.; Wei, W.; Hu, Y.; Kankanhalli, M.; Geng, W. Semi-Supervised Learning for Surface EMG-based Gesture Recognition. In Proceedings of the Twenty-Sixth International Joint Conference on Artificial Intelligence, IJCAI-17, Melbourne, Australia, 19–25 August 2017; pp. 1624–1630. [CrossRef]
26. Staudenmann, D.; Kingma, I.; Stegeman, D.; Van Dieen, J. Towards optimal multi-channel EMG electrode configurations in muscle force estimation: A high density EMG study. *J. Electromyogr. Kinesiol.* **2005**, *15*, 1–11. [CrossRef]
27. Atzori, M.; Gijsberts, A.; Heynen, S.; Mittaz Hager, A.G.; Deriaz, O.; Van Der Smagt, P.; Castellini, C.; Caputo, B.; Müller, H. Resource for the Biorobotics Community (Ninapro). In Proceedings of the IEEE International Conference on Biomedical Robotics and Biomechatronics, Rome, Italy, 24–27 June 2012.
28. Geng, W.; Du, Y.; Jin, W.; Wei, W.; Hu, Y.; Li, J. Gesture recognition by instantaneous surface EMG images. *Sci. Rep.* **2016**, *6*, 36571. [CrossRef]
29. Rojas-Martínez, M.; Mañanas, M.A.; Alonso, J.F. High-density surface EMG maps from upper-arm and forearm muscles. *Neuroeng. Rehabil.* **2012**, *9*, 85, [CrossRef]
30. Pizzolato, S.; Tagliapietra, L.; Cognolato, M.; Reggiani, M.; Müller, H.; Atzori, M. Comparison of six electromyography acquisition setups on hand movement classification tasks. *PLoS ONE* **2017**, *12*, e0186132. [CrossRef]
31. Oskoei, M.A.; Hu, H. Myoelectric control systems—A survey. *Biomed. Signal Process. Control* **2007**, *2*, 275–294. [CrossRef]
32. Atzori, M.; Cognolato, M.; Müller, H. Deep Learning with Convolutional Neural Networks Applied to Electromyography Data: A Resource for the Classification of Movements for Prosthetic Hands. *Front. Neurorobot.* **2016**, *10*, 9. [CrossRef]
33. Wang, K.J.; Tung, H.W.; Huang, Z.; Thakur, P.; Mao, Z.H.; You, M.X. EXGbuds: Universal Wearable Assistive Device for Disabled People to Interact with the Environment Seamlessly. In Proceedings of the HRI '18 Companion of the 2018 ACM/IEEE International Conference on Human-Robot Interaction, Chicago, IL, USA, 5–8 March 2018; pp. 369–370.
34. Bahdanau, D.; Cho, K.; Bengio, Y. Neural machine translation by jointly learning to align and translate. *arXiv* **2014**, arXiv:1409.0473.
35. Mikolov, T.; Karafiát, M.; Burget, L.; Černocký, J.; Khudanpur, S. Recurrent neural network based language model. In Proceedings of the 11th Annual Conference of the International Speech Communication Association, Makuhari, Chiba, Japan, 26–30 September 2010.

36. Hochreiter, S.; Schmidhuber, J. Long short-term memory. *Neural Comput.* **1997**, *9*, 1735–1780. [CrossRef]
37. Sutskever, I.; Vinyals, O.; Le, Q.V. Sequence to Sequence Learning with Neural Networks. In *Advances in Neural Information Processing Systems*; Neural Information Processing Systems Foundation, Inc.: Denver, CO, USA, 2014.
38. Cho, K.; Van Merriënboer, B.; Gulcehre, C.; Bahdanau, D.; Bougares, F.; Schwenk, H.; Bengio, Y. Learning Phrase Representations using RNN Encoder–Decoder for Statistical Machine Translation. In Proceedings of the Eighth Workshop on Syntax, Semantics and Structure in Statistical Translation, Doha, Qatar, 25 October 2014.
39. Yin, W.; Kann, K.; Yu, M.; Schütze, H. Comparative Study of CNN and RNN for Natural Language Processing. *CoRR* **2017**, arXiv:1702.01923.
40. Chung, J.; Gülçehre, Ç.; Cho, K.; Bengio, Y. Empirical Evaluation of Gated Recurrent Neural Networks on Sequence Modeling. *CoRR* **2014**, arXiv:1412.3555.
41. Van Dijk Johannes, P. High-density Surface EMG: Techniques and Applications at a Motor Unit Level. *Biocybern. Biomed. Eng.* **2012**, *32*, 3–27.
42. Guger, C.; Krausz, G.; Allison, B.; Edlinger, G. Comparison of Dry and Gel Based Electrodes for P300 Brain–Computer Interfaces. *Front. Neurosci.* **2012**, *6*, 60. [CrossRef]
43. Gonzalo Pomboza-Junez, J.H.T. *Hand Gesture Recognition Based on sEMG Signals Using Support Vector Machines*; Consumer Electronics: Berlin, Germany, 2016.
44. Allard, U.C.; Fall, C.L.; Drouin, A.; Campeau-Lecours, A.; Gosselin, C.; Glette, K.; Laviolette, F.; Gosselin, B. Deep Learning for Electromyographic Hand Gesture Signal Classification by Leveraging Transfer Learning. *CoRR* **2018**, arXiv:1801.07756.
45. Côté-Allard, U.; Fall, C.L.; Campeau-Lecours, A.; Gosselin, C.; Laviolette, F.; Gosselin, B. Transfer Learning for sEMG Hand Gestures Recognition Using Convolutional Neural Networks. In Proceedings of the IEEE International Conference on Systems, Banff, AB, Canada, 5–8 October 2017.
46. Adafruit. Myo Armband Teardown. 2016. Available online: https://learn.adafruit.com/myo-armband-teardown/inside-myo (accessed on 14 September 2018).
47. Farina, D.; Cescon, C.; Merletti, R. Influence of anatomical, physical, and detection-system parameters on surface EMG. *Biol. Cybern.* **2002**, *86*, 445–456. [CrossRef]
48. Kuiken, T.A.; Lowery, M.M.; Stoykov, N.S. The effect of subcutaneous fat on myoelectric signal amplitude and cross-talk. *Prosthet. Orthot. Int.* **2003**, *27*, 48–54. [CrossRef]
49. Ruder, S. An overview of gradient descent optimization algorithms. *CoRR* **2016**, arXiv:1609.04747.
50. Johnson, N.E.; Sowden, J.; Dilek, N.; Eichinger, K.; Burns, J.; Mcdermott, M.P.; Shy, M.E.; Herrmann, D.N. Prospective Study of Muscle Cramps in Charcot Marie Tooth Disease. *Muscle Nerve* **2015**, *51*, 485–488. [CrossRef]

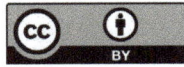

© 2019 by the authors. Licensee MDPI, Basel, Switzerland. This article is an open access article distributed under the terms and conditions of the Creative Commons Attribution (CC BY) license (http://creativecommons.org/licenses/by/4.0/).

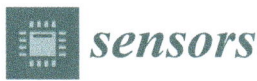

Article

Directional Forgetting for Stable Co-Adaptation in Myoelectric Control

Dennis Yeung [1,*], Dario Farina [2] and Ivan Vujaklija [1,*]

1. Department of Electrical Engineering and Automation, Aalto University, 02150 Espoo, Finland
2. Department of Bioengineering, Imperial College London, London SW7 2AZ, UK; d.farina@imperial.ac.uk
* Correspondence: dennis.yeung@aalto.fi (D.Y.); ivan.vujaklija@aalto.fi (I.V.)

Received: 12 April 2019; Accepted: 8 May 2019; Published: 13 May 2019

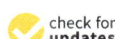

Abstract: Conventional myoelectric controllers provide a mapping between electromyographic signals and prosthetic functions. However, due to a number of instabilities continuously challenging this process, an initial mapping may require an extended calibration phase with long periods of user-training in order to ensure satisfactory performance. Recently, studies on co-adaptation have highlighted the benefits of concurrent user learning and machine adaptation where systems can cope with deficiencies in the initial model by learning from newly acquired data. However, the success remains highly dependent on careful weighting of these new data. In this study, we proposed a function driven directional forgetting approach to the recursive least-squares algorithm as opposed to the classic exponential forgetting scheme. By only discounting past information in the same direction of the new data, local corrections to the mapping would induce less distortion to other regions. To validate the approach, subjects performed a set of real-time myoelectric tasks over a range of forgetting factors. Results show that directional forgetting with a forgetting factor of 0.995 outperformed exponential forgetting as well as unassisted user learning. Moreover, myoelectric control remained stable after adaptation with directional forgetting over a range of forgetting factors. These results indicate that a directional approach to discounting past training data can improve performance and alleviate sensitivities to parameter selection in recursive adaptation algorithms.

Keywords: co-adaptation; directional forgetting; electromyography; myoelectric control; upper-limb prostheses

1. Introduction

Surface electromyography (EMG) offers a non-invasive window to the peripheral nervous system (PNS) and has been used as the control input for powered prostheses since the 1950s [1,2]. In particular, myoelectric devices have been marketed towards upper-limb amputees with the appeal of providing partial functional restoration of the affected limb whilst retaining anthropomorphic aesthetics. However, most clinically available devices still employ a simplified control scheme which restricts operation to highly unintuitive sequential activation of degrees-of-freedom (DoF). Contractions from an agonist–antagonist muscle pair drives device operation along one DoF while mode-switching to other DoFs is toggled via co-contraction or pulsing [3].

More sophisticated interpretations of residual muscle activity based on pattern-recognition (PR) have since been investigated [4]. Using features (in time or frequency domain, or a combination of both) extracted from multi-channel EMG data, a repertoire of analytically distinguishable contraction patterns can be learned by the system. This allows amputees to access different prosthetic functions without switching modes while controlling actuation speeds based on contraction intensities. This control scheme has been shown to require lower cognitive load to operate and outperforms traditional direct control in online tests [5,6]. Despite these reported advantages, PR control is ultimately inconsistent with natural limb function [7]. While natural movements rely on concurrent actuation over multiple DoFs, the discrete output approximations offered by PR restricts prosthesis control to sequential operations. Simultaneous DoF activations can in principle be achieved by increasing the number of classes trained or by employing multiple classifiers in various topologies [8,9], but these methods compromise on classification accuracy and system scalability [10].

These drawbacks pertaining to the lack of simultaneous control are addressed in regression-based methods. By relying on a continuous mapping between EMG feature space and prosthesis function, simultaneous and proportional control (SPC) over multiple DoFs is enabled [7]. Such a mapping between residual muscle activations and controller output can be established by regressing the EMG characteristics of phantom limb commands to either the mirrored kinematics of the healthy limb [11,12], or to the position of a virtual cursor cueing the phantom movements [13–15].

In contrast to PR, where changes in muscle activation strategies can only be noticed when a decision boundary between classes is already crossed, a continuous mapping employed by regressors provides uninterrupted feedback. As such, regression-based controllers are more responsive to user adaptation as corrective measures are immediately reflected [16]. For this reason, users can partly compensate for artificially induced signal non-stationarities when using a regression-based control, contrary to a PR-based controller [17]. This characteristic is particularly advantages as environmental factors are known to perturb signal statistics. Muscle fatigue, perspiration, electrode displacement and even limb positioning contribute to the non-stationarity of recorded EMG resulting in the gradual deterioration of controller performance [18–20]. Although user adaptation allows partial compensation for these effects, it is thought that adaptive systems can offer a more robust and less cognitively demanding solution. Such systems learn from newly acquired data as the old model becomes defective. However, this has mostly been studied with PR-based controllers [21–27] and there are only a few examples of adaptive regression-based controllers [28–30]. In both cases, machine adaptation may occur either concurrently with user adaptation in real-time or can be implemented as incremental steps in learning.

Recently, Hahne et al. demonstrated improved myoelectric control performance with congenital amputees through a co-adaptive learning approach using recursive least squares [29]. However, adaptation stability is shown to be highly sensitive to the forgetting factor. Adaptation with certain forgetting rates results in "estimator wind-up" [31] where past data are discarded in such a way that the model overfits to new training data. In the most severe cases, this has resulted in subjects losing the ability to navigate the majority of the solution space. Various solutions to this challenge have been proposed in the form of time-varying forgetting factors [32] as well forgetting that is non-uniform in space [33]. With the latter approach, only past data in the direction of new data are discounted, meaning that only obsolete and replaceable information is forgotten.

In this study, we hypothesised that the overall performance and the instability issues encountered using the classic exponential forgetting scheme can be addressed by implementing a directional forgetting scheme. This was verified experimentally by conducting online evaluations of co-adaptation efficiency and stability with directional forgetting over a wide range of forgetting factors. Classic exponential forgetting using the generalised best performing forgetting factor reported in [29] was also tested, allowing for comparisons to be drawn.

2. Materials and Methods

2.1. Subjects

Five able-bodied subjects with no prior experience of myoelectric control participated in the study: one left-hand dominant, female, aged 20 and four right-hand dominant subjects, two female and two male aged 22–27. All subjects gave their written informed consent. This study was performed in compliance with the Declaration of Helsinki and approved by the Imperial College Research Ethics Committee in London, UK (ICREC ref:18IC4685).

2.2. Setup and Data Acquisition

During the experiments, subjects were seated in front of a monitor with both arms relaxed by their sides. 16 monopolar sEMG channels were acquired using pre-gelled electrodes (Neuroline® 720, Ambu, Denmark) placed around their dominant forearm in two rings. The electrode centres of the proximal ring were located approximately 3 cm below the lateral epicondyle of the elbow while the distal ring was adjacent just below. Horizontal distances between the centres of adjacent electrodes ranged 2.5–3.5 cm depending on the size of the subject's forearm. Two additional gelled electrodes were attached just above the wrist of the dominant arm near the radial and ulnar styloid processes as references for the pre-amplifier and bio-amplifier. This configuration allowed for SPC over two DoFs without the need for targeted electrode placement and was aligned to that of past studies involving SPC where electrode placement is not targeted [15,16,29,34,35] and an example can be seen in Figure 1.

The detected signals were pre-amplified by five and then further amplified with a gain of either 500 or 1000 (amplifier EMGUSB2+, OT Bioelettronica, Italy), and sampled at 2048 Hz. The amplifier filtered the signals in the 10–500 Hz band. All subsequent software functionalities including signal processing, offline training and online testing were carried out using a custom MATLAB-based framework.

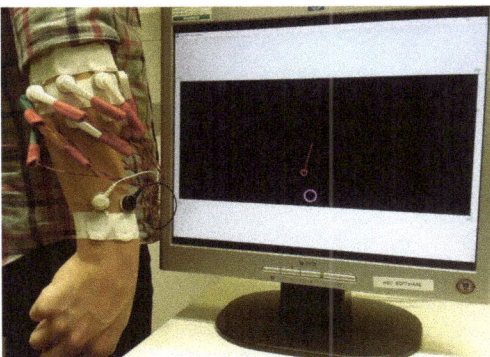

Figure 1. Experimental setup showing electrode position and visual feedback of the virtual task space. The red cursor is controlled via the myoelectric interface while the pink circle represents the target.

The acquired data were treated to adaptive common average filtering [36] and a fifth-order Butterworth band-pass filter with cut-offs at 20 Hz and 500 Hz [37]. Finally, a notch filter centred at 50 Hz was used to remove line noise. The filtered EMG data were processed in windows of 160 ms length that progressed in steps of 40 ms (120 ms of overlap) and the RMS values of each channel in the window were extracted as features.

2.3. Linear Regression

SPC can be achieved using a basic linear regression (LR) where the predicted output command, across a number of DoFs, is calculated as the instantaneous linear mixture of the input features:

$$\hat{\mathbf{y}}(t) = \mathbf{W}^\mathsf{T}\mathbf{x}(t) \quad (1)$$

where $\hat{\mathbf{y}}(t)$ is a column vector with each element corresponding to a single DoF, $\mathbf{W}$ is a weight matrix and $\mathbf{x}(t)$ is the input feature vector. Initialisation of this model involves finding the matrix $\mathbf{W}$ which minimises the sum-squared errors of training samples, as shown in Equation (2), where the batch nature of model initialisation has been reflected with sample number n. This was found analytically using the Moore–Penrose pseudo-inverse method shown in Equation (3).

$$\epsilon = \sum_{n=1}^{N}(\mathbf{y}(n) - \mathbf{W}^\mathsf{T}\mathbf{x}(n))^2 \tag{2}$$

$$\mathbf{W} = (\mathbf{XX}^\mathsf{T})^{-1}\mathbf{XY}^\mathsf{T} \tag{3}$$

A biasing input was also incorporated to allow for an offset of the solution plane and, as such, $\mathbf{x}(t)$ is prepended with a unity element and W is expanded with an additional row. Hence, $\mathbf{Y}$ is a $\langle M \times N \rangle$ matrix of target labels (visual cue coordinates) and $\mathbf{X}$ is a matrix of training features of dimensions $\langle (C+1) \times N \rangle$. M denotes the number of controllable DoFs, C is the number of EMG channels and N is the number of training samples. The instantaneous estimation of the command output (before post-processing) is simply obtained by solving Equation (1).

2.4. Recursive Least Squares with Exponential Forgetting

To facilitate model adaptation in real-time, the batch method of Equation (3) needs to be resolved. However, this is resource intensive due to the linear scaling of computational complexity with the number of training samples. Here, the recursive least-squares (RLS) algorithm may be deployed instead. Namely, as new data are obtained, the algorithm utilises past results to efficiently compute an updated least-squares estimation of the regression model parameters [31]. RLS with exponential forgetting (RLS-EF) extends the algorithm by exponentially discounting past data with each update, thus allowing for new system dynamics to override old data. This is done via the inclusion of a forgetting factor λ to the cost function in Equation (2), resulting in:

$$\epsilon = \sum_{t=0}^{T} \lambda^{T-t}(\mathbf{y}(t) - \mathbf{W}^\mathsf{T}\mathbf{x}(t))^2 \tag{4}$$

where the notation of sample number n has been replaced with time t to reflect online implementation. Smaller values of λ correspond to a heavier discounting of past data while a value of 1 gives the "growing window" RLS algorithm where all data, new and old, are equally weighted.

The following set of update equations may then be executed to optimise the cost function (Equation (4)) as new data become available:

$$\mathbf{a}(t) = \mathbf{y}^\mathsf{T}(t) - \mathbf{x}^\mathsf{T}(t)\mathbf{W}(t) \tag{5}$$

$$\mathbf{g}(t) = \mathbf{P}(t-1)\mathbf{x}(t)(\lambda + \mathbf{x}^\mathsf{T}(t)\lambda^{-1}\mathbf{P}(t-1))^{-1} \tag{6}$$

$$\mathbf{P}(t) = \lambda^{-1}\mathbf{P}^\mathsf{T}(t-1) - \mathbf{g}(t)\mathbf{x}^\mathsf{T}(t)\lambda^{-1}\mathbf{P}(t-1) \tag{7}$$

$$\mathbf{W}(t+1) = \mathbf{W}(t) + \mathbf{a}(t)\mathbf{g}(t) \tag{8}$$

The initial weight matrix $\mathbf{W}(0)$ is given by the batch method of Equation (3) while the exponentially weighted inverse of the sample covariance matrix $\mathbf{P}(0)$, is initialised as $(\mathbf{XX}^\mathsf{T})^{-1}$.

With each iteration of the update rules, past data retained in the information matrix $\mathbf{R}(t) = \mathbf{P}(t)^{-1}$ are uniformly down-scaled by λ and updated with new data $(\mathbf{x}(t)\mathbf{x}(t)^\mathsf{T})$:

$$\mathbf{R}(t+1) = \lambda \mathbf{R}(t) + \mathbf{x}(t)\mathbf{x}^\mathsf{T}(t) \tag{9}$$

2.5. Recursive Least Squares with Directional Forgetting

As an alternative to exponential forgetting, RLS can be implemented in such a way as to employ a more content related forgetting scheme. As presented in [38], selective forgetting in the direction of the new input is achieved by the decomposition of the information matrix, $\mathbf{R}(t)$, into $\mathbf{R}_1(t)$, which represents old data that are orthogonal to the new data, and $\mathbf{R}_2(t)$, which represents old data to be discounted:

$$\mathbf{R}(t) = \mathbf{R}_1(t) + \mathbf{R}_2(t) \tag{10}$$

$$\mathbf{R}_1(t)\mathbf{x}(t) = 0, \ \mathbf{x}(t) \neq 0 \tag{11}$$

$$\mathbf{R}_2(t)\mathbf{x}(t) = \mathbf{R}(t)\mathbf{x}(t) \tag{12}$$

$$\mathbf{R}(t+1) = \mathbf{R}_1(t) + \lambda \mathbf{R}_2(t) + \mathbf{x}(t)\mathbf{x}^\mathsf{T}(t) \tag{13}$$

With Equations (10)–(12), $\mathbf{R}_1(t)$ and $\mathbf{R}_2(t)$ are not yet fully defined, however, as the new data are only of rank 1. A fair requirement would be that $\mathbf{R}_2(t)$ should also be of rank 1 with the rank of $\mathbf{R}_1(t)$ as C (C + 1 is the order of $\mathbf{R}(t)$). With the inclusion of these constraints, a unique solution for both matrices may be found. Effecting this decomposition to the recursive algorithm gives the new update Equations (14)–(17):

$$\mathbf{a}(t) = \mathbf{y}^\mathsf{T}(t) - \mathbf{x}^\mathsf{T}\mathbf{W}(t) \tag{14}$$

$$\bar{\mathbf{P}} = \mathbf{P}(t-1) + \frac{1-\lambda}{\lambda} \frac{\mathbf{x}(t)\mathbf{x}^\mathsf{T}(t)}{\mathbf{x}^\mathsf{T}(t)\mathbf{P}^{-1}(t-1)\mathbf{x}(t)} \tag{15}$$

$$\mathbf{P}(t) = \bar{\mathbf{P}} - \frac{\bar{\mathbf{P}}\mathbf{x}(t)\mathbf{x}^\mathsf{T}(t)\bar{\mathbf{P}}(t)}{1 + \mathbf{x}^\mathsf{T}(t)\bar{\mathbf{P}}(t)\mathbf{x}(t)} \tag{16}$$

$$\mathbf{W}(t+1) = \mathbf{W}(t) + \mathbf{P}(t)\mathbf{x}(t)\mathbf{a}^\mathsf{T}(t) \tag{17}$$

2.6. Calibration Phase

Each experiment started with the calibration phase during which training data for the base LR model were collected. Subjects performed three repetitions of single DoF motions that corresponded to a visual cue shown on the monitor. Starting from the centre of the task space, the cue first travelled to the right of the screen, stayed for 1.5 s then returned to the origin after which it travelled to the left of the screen and dwelled for another 1.5 s before moving back to the origin. These horizontal movements were executed three times, after which three repetitions of the same nature were preformed in the vertical directions. During these cue movements, subjects were asked to match the horizontal displacement of the cue proportionally by performing wrist flexion/extension, and match vertical displacements with wrist abduction/adduction. The baseline regression model was then obtained using the batch initialisation method described in Section 2.3.

2.7. Online Myocontrol

Once regression models were trained, the online myocontrol portion of the experiment started, during which, subjects were able to manoeuvre a cursor in a virtual task space. Cursor position was initially estimated from Equation (1) with additional post-processing to improve controller performance.

Since no kinematic or kinetic measurements were taken as labels during the calibration phase, the mappings obtained from the initial open-looped training tended to be under-scaled. Each direction was therefore boosted:

$$\begin{bmatrix}\hat{y}'_1(t)\\\hat{y}'_2(t)\end{bmatrix} = \begin{bmatrix}\tau_{1a}\hat{y}_1(t)\\\tau_{2b}\hat{y}_2(t)\end{bmatrix} \tag{18}$$

where: $\begin{cases}a=1, & \hat{y}_1(t) \geq 0\\a=2, & \hat{y}_1(t) < 0\end{cases}$ & $\begin{cases}b=1, & \hat{y}_2(t) \geq 0\\b=2, & \hat{y}_2(t) < 0\end{cases}$ \qquad(19)

Here, different gains were applied depending on the sign of the estimated horizontal (DoF 1) cursor displacement (τ_{11} and τ_{12} for positive and negative displacement, respectively). Likewise, different gains were applied for positive and negative vertical (DoF 2) estimates of the cursor (τ_{21} and τ_{22}, respectively). All gains were tuned manually after the calibration phase to ensure effortless coverage of the task space. The criterion for setting gain values required subjects to be able to comfortably displace the cursor by 90 density-independent pixels (dp) in all single and combined DoF activations.

Finally, a seventh-order moving-average filter was applied, giving the post-processed controller output $\hat{y}''(t)$. The filter was implemented to reduce endpoint jitter and effectively smoothen the cursor movement.

2.8. Evaluation Runs

To gauge myoelectric control performance, target reaching exercises were conducted. Each run involved manoeuvring a cursor towards a sequence of 16 target circles with radii of 8 dp inside a task space that was 400 × 180 dp (target was <0.3% of the task space). The targets were evenly distributed in an inner and outer ring. Targets of the inner ring lied 40 dp from the origin while the outer ring had a radius of 75 dp with all targets evenly distributed about the origin to ensure a mixture of tasks requiring single and various degrees of simultaneous DoF control.

Subjects were given 10 s to complete each task and to successfully do so the cursor had to dwell within the target for 0.5 s. Between each task, subjects were prompted to relax and let the cursor return to the task space origin before the next task was presented. The sequence of targets presented to each subject was randomised across runs.

2.9. Adaptation Runs

Concurrent adaptation of algorithm and user took place during adaptation runs where subjects attempted target reaching exercises similar to those in the evaluation runs described in the previous section. However, if the task had not been completed after 5 s, then the mapping was deemed deficient and machine adaptation was triggered. System adaptation was driven by the execution of the update rules described in Sections 2.4 and 2.5, in which the target position and input EMG features were used to update the regression model such that the cursor converged towards the target. Machine adaptation was ceased when either the target had been reached or the task execution time had expired. A schematic of this closed-loop adaptive myoelectric controller is illustrated in Figure 2.

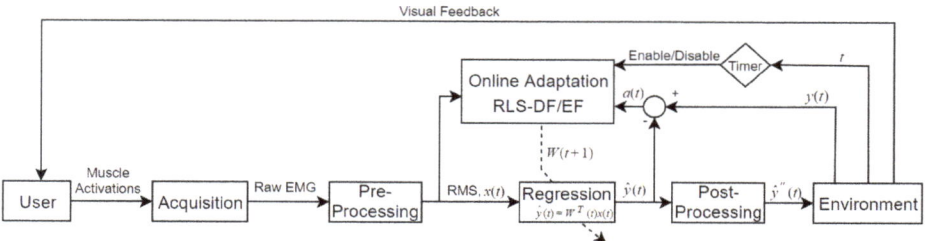

Figure 2. Online estimation and adaptation schematic. During adaptation runs, online adaptation with RLS was triggered if the current target was not reached within 5 s. The dotted diagonal line striking through the controller block (Regression) indicates conditional parameter update.

2.10. Run Sequence

The experiment consisted of 12 consecutive runs, which were a mixture of evaluation and adaptation runs. The sequence of assessments is shown in Figure 3. Run 1 (Baseline) was an evaluation run which gauged the baseline performance of the subject. Subsequently, the effects of machine adaptation were tested in the next 10 runs using RLS-DF using λ ranging from 0.995–0.93 and RLS-EF with $\lambda = 0.995$. This was done by alternating sequences of adaptation runs (Runs 2, 4, 6, 8 and 10) and evaluations runs (Runs 3, 5, 7, 9 and 11). During an adaptation run, system adaptation was enabled with the forgetting factor and RLS variant to be tested. Each adaptation run was followed by an evaluation run. which tested the performance of the adapted model. Between each adaptation/evaluation run pair, the regression model was reverted back to the original, batch-trained condition. This was repeated until all the forgetting factors of the RLS-DF and the RLS-EF had been tested. The order of which these were tested was randomised across subjects to prevent biasing of results. The final test, Run 12 (User Learning), was an evaluation run using the base regression model which provided a reference for how much performance gain can be attributed to inherent skill improvement of the user.

Subjects were informed about the inclusion of machine adaptation prior to the adaptation runs, although no information pertaining to the actual mechanism was provided. Furthermore, pilot experiments had shown significant increases in performance by subjects between the first and second run due to the effects of learning. As such, prior to the commencement of the block of runs described earlier, a training evaluation run was conducted. This allowed participants to become familiar with myoelectric control and the virtual testing environment.

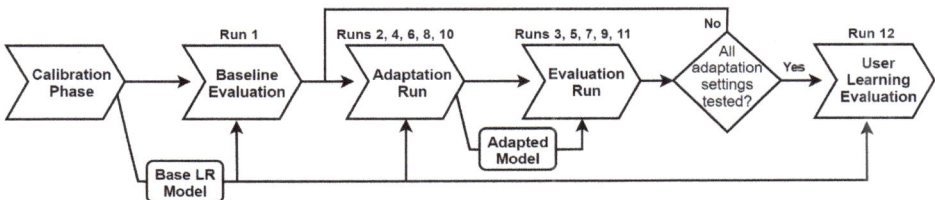

Figure 3. Flow diagram of the experimental procedure. The adaptation settings that were tested include: RLS-DF with $\lambda = 0.995, 0.97, 0.95$, and 0.93, and RLS-EF with $\lambda = 0.995$. The order of adaptation settings tested was randomised for each subject to prevent biasing of results.

2.11. Performance Metrics

Four metrics were implemented to quantify each subject's performance across the runs and such metrics have been used in past studies on myoelectric control [15,16,34]. The Completion Rate (CR) of each run is the ratio between the number of targets reached and the total number of targets. Completion Time (CT) shows the time needed to reach each individual target, Path Efficiency (PE) indicates the ratio between the optimal path from the origin to the target (straight line distance) and the actual trajectory of the cursor. Throughput (TP) is used to measure the information transfer capabilities of the human-machine interface and is calculated from a task's index of difficulty (ID) and completion time:

$$TP = \frac{ID}{CT} \quad (20)$$

This measure is based on Shannon's Extension of Fitt's Law, as presented in [39], with ID expressed as a relationship between target displacement in DoFs 1 and 2 (D_1, D_2) and target radius (W):

$$ID = log_2 \left(\frac{(0.5D_1 + 0.5D_2)^2}{W} + 1 \right) \quad (21)$$

2.12. Statistical Analysis

To determine the co-adaptation stability of RLS-DF over a range of forgetting factors, the significance of performance differences between runs was calculated for all appropriate metrics. Values of TP, CT and PE for all targets were subjected to a two-way mixed ANOVA where the between-target factor was subject and the within-target factor was adaptation setting. The levels of adaptation setting include

Baseline and User Learning (Runs 1 and 12, respectively) as well as RLS-DF($\lambda = 0.93$), RLS-DF($\lambda = 0.95$), RLS-DF($\lambda = 0.97$), RLS-DF($\lambda = 0.995$) and RLS-EF($\lambda = 0.995$) (randomised amongst Runs 3, 5, 7, 9 and 11). Results from adaptation runs were not included in the analysis, as convergence to targets during those runs were machine-aided.

In the case where there was no significant interaction between the factors, the main effects were reported. If significant interaction was detected, focused Friedman Tests were conducted across subjects to detect the presence of simple effects. If the test revealed statistically significant differences between the adaptation settings, pairwise comparisons were done using the Dunn–Bonferroni test.

2.13. Adaptation Analysis

The resultant model from each adaptation run was compared to its base model. Changes to the model weights of the LR-based mappings were quantified using dot products between the normalised row vectors of the original model and the adapted model. A result of 1 represents no change in the contribution of the corresponding EMG channel to each DoF activation while a value of 0 represents a completely orthogonal DoF activation. The averaged dot-product value was then used to indicate the degree to which the original model was altered through online adaptation.

3. Results

The overall performance results are shown in Figure 4. Two-way mixed ANOVA was conducted for TP, CT and PE. Mixed ANOVA assumes equal variances between the categories of the between-targets factor (subject) at each level of the within-targets factor (adaptation setting). This was assessed using the modified Levene's Test for Homogeneity of variance [40] with all metrics meeting this criterion ($p > 0.05$). Variances of the differences between the levels of the repeated-measures factor was checked using Mauchly's Test of Sphericity. Both CT ($p = 0.371$) and PE ($p = 0.099$) satisfied this assumption but TP ($p = 0.009$) failed; therefore, the Greenhouse–Geisser correction was applied to the analysis of TP.

Results from the mixed ANOVA's indicated significant interaction between adaptation settings and subjects for all metrics (TP: $F(20.925, 392.340) = 2.039$, $p = 0.005$; CT: $F(24, 450)$ 2.293, $p = 0.001$; PE: $F(24, 450) = 1.979$, $p = 0.004$). As Shapiro–Wilk tests indicated non-normality of some results, the validity of interaction differences were confirmed by conducting the same testing on square-root transformations of the data which resulted in normality. As the study was mainly concerned with the adaptation stability of different forgetting factors, only the simple main effect of adaptation setting was investigated. For every subject, statistical difference between adaptation settings was checked with the Friedman Test. In the case of significance, Dunn–Bonferonni post-hoc tests were conducted with results highlighted in Figure 4. Significant differences spread across all performance metrics and all subjects except Subject 1 were detected. This occurred between "Baseline" and RLS-DF with $\lambda = 0.93$ and 0.995, RLS-EF with $\lambda = 0.995$ and "User Learning". However, no significance was found in the differences between the forgetting factors of RLS-DF.

No statistical testing was conducted for CR as the number of samples for each adaptation setting was limited to one per subject. As shown in Figure 5a, RLS-DF with $\lambda = 0.995$ (0.85 ± 0.13) was the best performer on average followed by RLS-EF($\lambda = 0.995$) (0.80 ± 0.14). While all online-adapted models performed better compared to the initial evaluation with the batch-trained model (Baseline) (0.51 ± 0.12), performance with the same model at the end of testing "User Learning" (0.74 ± 0.16) made the online adaptation with RLS-DF, $\lambda = 0.97$ (0.64 ± 0.17), $\lambda = 0.95$ (0.63 ± 0.17) and $\lambda = 0.93$ (0.70 ± 0.15) obsolete.

Quantification of model adaptation based on dot products is shown in Figure 5b. Here, RLS-EF was shown to induce the most changes to the model with the lowest average dot product of 0.65 and the largest standard deviation of ± 0.21. Within RLS-DF, adaptation with $\lambda = 0.995$ resulted in the largest changes to the weights with a mean of 0.86 ± 0.08 while $\lambda = 0.97$ showed the least change and spread with 0.96 ± 0.03.

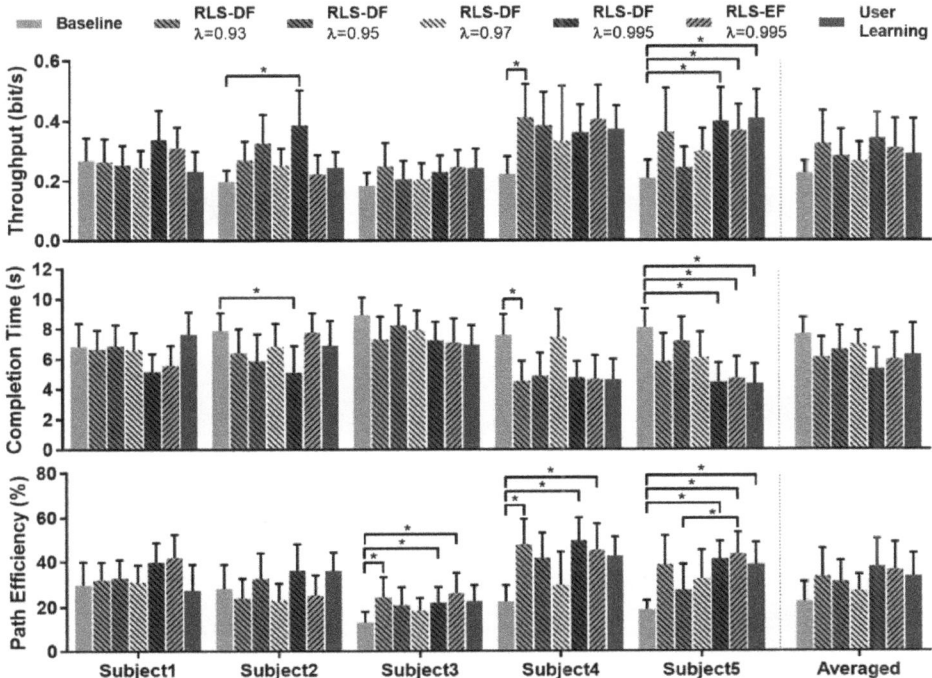

Figure 4. Results from the evaluation of the five subjects. * indicates statistical significance detected with Dunn–Bonferroni pairwise testing.

Adaptation with RLS-DF ($\lambda = 0.995$) produced models that yielded the best TP result averaged across all subjects (0.34 ± 0.06 bits/s). Similarly, RLS-DF with $\lambda = 0.995$ produced the best overall results for CT (5.35 ± 0.98 s) and PE (37.75 ± 8.96%), as shown on the right-side panel of Figure 4. In comparison, the averaged TP, CT and PE results for RLS-EF with $\lambda = 0.995$ were 0.31 ± 0.07 bits/s, 5.97 ± 1.26 s and 36.48 ± 8.78% respectively. Overall, RLS-DF with $\lambda = 0.995$ was demonstrated to perform best in all metrics and consistently surpassed the results of RLS-EF.

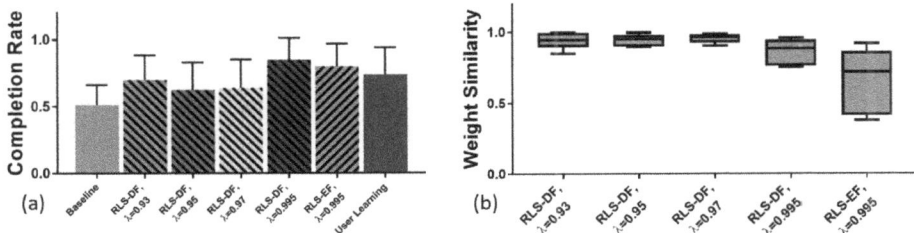

Figure 5. (a) Completion ratio of evaluation runs. Runs involving machine and user co-adaptation, regardless of algorithm or forgetting factor, had, on average, higher target hit rates compared to initial evaluations with the batch-trained model (Baseline). (b) Averaged dot products between normalised row vectors of weights from batch-trained models and their online-adapted versions. A value of 1 indicates no change to the sensitivities of the mapping while lower values represent larger changes to the model during machine adaptation.

4. Discussion

Directional forgetting was proposed to improve the myoelectric performance and stability of classic co-adaptive RLS algorithm. This was experimentally verified when evaluation runs of RLS-DF over a wide range of forgetting factors showed no significant decrease in performance for all subjects tested. Since the experimental set-up and timing scheme were similar to the original study by Hahne et al. on co-adaptation with RLS-EF, direct comparisons can be made between the performance of RLS-DF and the results obtained in [29] using RLS-EF. One of the most noticeable improvements then was RLS-DF's prevention of severe over-fitting of the mapping to the target most recently adapted towards. Even with the most aggressive forgetting factor of $\lambda = 0.93$, RLS-DF did not induce a complete loss in the ability to navigate the solution space (example in Figure 6), as was reported to occur with RLS-EF at $\lambda = 0.96$.

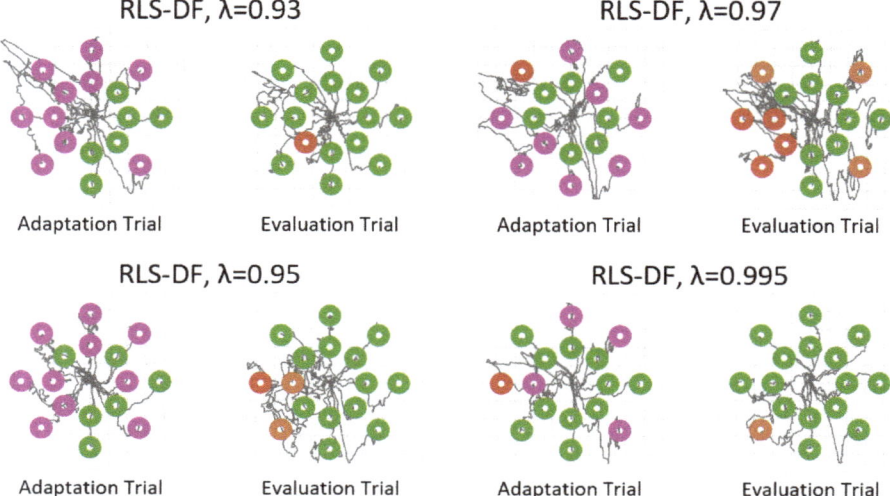

Figure 6. Cursor trajectories of adaptation and evaluation runs with RLS-DF from Subject 4. Green circles represent targets that were successfully reached, orange circles represent targets that were hit but dwell time was insufficient and red circles represent targets that were not hit within the time limit. Purple circles are only present in adaptation runs and represent targets that were reached with the aid of machine adaptation. Though some forgetting factors performed better than others, it can be observed that the solution space is still navigable after adaptation regardless of λ.

When past data were uniformly forgotten, large changes were induced in the mappings, as highlighted in the model weights analyses. Here, adaptation with RLS-EF induced the most amount of change with regards to how each input element contributed to the activation of DoFs in the virtual task space. Conversely, selective discounting of past data allowed for subtler updating of model parameters, which improved stability and yielded better performance. A relatable conclusion was made in Courad et al.'s study [30], where localised and modulated updating of muscle pulling vectors in a virtual biomechanics-based model resulted in faster and more stable co-adaptative performances against perturbations when compared to co-adaptation with fixed global gains.

It is worth noting that subjects consistently performed worse in the evaluations of RLS-DF co-adaptation with $\lambda = 0.93$ and 0.995. One would expect, instead, a peak in performance indicating an optimal forgetting factor with performance dropping as λ deviates from the optimal value. Conversely, experimental results show a drop in performance at moderate values of λ. A potential explanation may be that those values of λ represent adaptation which is neither aggressive nor slow enough.

Given that the study set an arbitrary time limit of 5 s to deem machine adaptation as necessary for reaching a target, this may also be the time when a user would decide to discard current activation strategies in lieu of more exploratory strategies to reach the target. With an aggressive rate of machine adaptation, the user would observe a faster automatic convergence of the cursor to the target, thus, abandoning their own exploration. With more passive machine adaptation, the online mapping of exploratory activations to the target would be far less destructive while automatic convergence of the cursor to the target is still occurring. As such, this also highlights an important flaw in the current approach taken where all input is directly assigned to the target during online adaptation without regard for true user intent.

While Hahne et al. emphasised how this co-adaptation technique is well suited for enhancing the initial batch training for amputees who may experience difficulty generating combined DoF activations [29], signal non-stationarities remain a primary cause for performance degradation. Hence, future work may investigate the robustness of RLS-DF co-adaptation under non-stationary environments.

Long-term stability of myocontrol with machine adaptation was, in part, investigated by Gijberts et al. [28] who conducted offline finger force estimation in a multi-session experiment. Of particular note was the inclusion of a practical incremental learning scheme that can be initiated by the user. They used visual cues as training labels during adaptation, forgoing the need for measurement equipment. While absolute performance was inferior to closed-loop adaptation with measured ground truths, degradation was nonetheless curbed. This then raises the question of how RLS-DF adaptation for position control may perform in a similar context, where adaptation can be triggered by the user and new data labelled from visual cues are used to enable open-loop adaptation on-demand. However, in this case, machine adaptation would be incremental rather than concurrent.

The complications of mislabelling exploratory activations or providing accurate ground truths for machine adaptation can be circumnavigated by unsupervised methods [23]. Past works have shown promising results of extracting basis synergies for SPC through blind factorisation of EMG into the appropriate number ranks using non-negative factorisation (NMF) [10,34]. More recently, Lin et al. [35] demonstrated that imposing sparseness constraints to latent control primitives allows for basis information to be extracted from simultaneous DoFs activations which opens up the possibility for adaptation during arbitrary activations.

Thus far, this study indicated improved co-adaptation outcomes from implementing directional forgetting. However, further work needs to be done to truly validate the benefits of this approach with regards to actual prosthesis performance. For this claim to be made, a more rigorous study would have to be conducted involving the participation of actual end-users (amputees) performing real-world tasks. Indeed, the abstracted VR-based assessment implemented here lacks accurate representation of the physical constraints of prosthetic devices. As such, future developments would include optimisation of this approach such that it can be implemented as part of the process leading to prosthetic device use. While integration of this co-adaptive paradigm to the use of hand prostheses has already been done in [14], the study itself does not try to quantify the benefits of the co-adaptation procedure to prosthesis use.

5. Conclusions

This study experimentally demonstrated, on a small number of volunteers, that a more principled approach to discarding obsolete training data (RLS-DF) improves performance and co-adaptation stability over previously tested methods. Online implementation and VR based control allowed subjects to embrace the adaptive nature of the system and surpass pure user learning. However, the true advantages of the approach will be investigated in the future when a number of limb impaired participants will be recruited with an idea to test the system using a fully fitted prosthetic device. Given that the presented algorithmic extension retains a recursive nature, it remains suitable for embedded deployment and, therefore, clinical translation.

Author Contributions: Conceptualisation, D.Y., D.F. and I.V.; Methodology, D.Y., D.F. and I.V.; Software, D.Y. and I.V.; Validation, D.Y.; Formal Analysis, D.Y.; Investigation, D.Y. and I.V.; Resources, D.F. and I.V.; Data Curation, D.Y.; Writing—Original Draft Preparation, D.Y., D.F. and I.V.; Writing—Review and Editing, D.Y., D.F. and I.V.; Visualisation, D.Y. and I.V.; Supervision, D.F. and I.V.; Project Administration, D.F. and I.V.; and Funding acquisition, D.F. and I.V.

Funding: Research was supported by the European Union's Horizon 2020 research and innovation program under grant agreement number 687795 (project INPUT).

Conflicts of Interest: The authors declare no conflict of interest.

References

1. Battye, C.K.; Nightingale, A.; Whillis, J. The Use of Meyo-electric Currents in the Operation of Prostheses. *J. Bone Joint Surg.* **1955**, *37*, 506–510. [CrossRef]
2. Bottomley, A.H. Myo-Electric Control of Powered Prostheses. *J. Bone Joint Surg.* **1965**, *47*, 411–415. [CrossRef]
3. Vujaklija, I.; Farina, D.; Aszmann, O. New developments in prosthetic arm systems. *Orthop. Res. Rev.* **2016**, *8*, 31–39. [CrossRef] [PubMed]
4. Scheme, E.; Englehart, K. Electromyogram pattern recognition for control of powered upper-limb prostheses: State of the art and challenges for clinical use. *J. Rehabil. Res. Dev.* **2011**, *48*, 643–660. [CrossRef]
5. Wurth, S.M.; Hargrove, L.J. A real-time comparison between direct control, sequential pattern recognition control and simultaneous pattern recognition control using a Fitts' law style assessment procedure. *J. NeuroEng. Rehabil.* **2014**. [CrossRef]
6. Zhang, W.; White, M.; Zahabi, M.; Winslow, A.T.; Zhang, F.; Huang, H.; Kaber, D. Cognitive workload in conventional direct control vs. pattern recognition control of an upper-limb prosthesis. In Proceedings of the 2016 IEEE International Conference on Systems, Man, and Cybernetics (SMC), Budapest, Hungary, 9–12 October 2016; pp. 002335–002340. [CrossRef]
7. Jiang, N.; Dosen, S.; Muller, K.R.; Farina, D. Myoelectric Control of Artificial Limbs—Is There a Need to Change Focus? [In the Spotlight]. *IEEE Signal Process. Mag.* **2012**, *29*, 152–150. [CrossRef]
8. Young, A.J.; Smith, L.H.; Rouse, E.J.; Hargrove, L.J. Classification of Simultaneous Movements Using Surface EMG Pattern Recognition. *IEEE Trans. Biomed. Eng.* **2013**, *60*, 1250–1258. [CrossRef]
9. Ortiz-Catalan, M.; Hkansson, B.; Brnemark, R. Real-Time and Simultaneous Control of Artificial Limbs Based on Pattern Recognition Algorithms. *IEEE Trans. Neural Syst. Rehabil. Eng.* **2014**, *22*, 756–764. [CrossRef] [PubMed]
10. Jiang, N.; Englehart, K.; Parker, P. Extracting Simultaneous and Proportional Neural Control Information for Multiple-DOF Prostheses From the Surface Electromyographic Signal. *IEEE Trans. Biomed. Eng.* **2009**, *56*, 1070–1080. [CrossRef]
11. Jiang, N.; Vest-Nielsen, J.L.; Muceli, S.; Farina, D. EMG-based simultaneous and proportional estimation of wrist/hand kinematics in uni-lateral trans-radial amputees. *J. NeuroEng. Rehabil.* **2012**, *9*, 42. [CrossRef]
12. Muceli, S.; Farina, D. Simultaneous and Proportional Estimation of Hand Kinematics From EMG During Mirrored Movements at Multiple Degrees-of-Freedom. *IEEE Trans. Neural Syst. Rehabil. Eng.* **2012**, *20*, 371–378. [CrossRef]
13. Ameri, A.; Kamavuako, E.N.; Scheme, E.J.; Englehart, K.B.; Parker, P.A. Real-time, simultaneous myoelectric control using visual target-based training paradigm. *Biomed. Signal Process. Control* **2014**, *13*, 8–14. [CrossRef]
14. Hahne, J.M.; Schweisfurth, M.A.; Koppe, M.; Farina, D. Simultaneous control of multiple functions of bionic hand prostheses: Performance and robustness in end users. *Sci. Robot.* **2018**, *3*, eaat3630. [CrossRef]
15. Vujaklija, I.; Shalchyan, V.; Kamavuako, E.N.; Jiang, N.; Marateb, H.R.; Farina, D. Online mapping of EMG signals into kinematics by autoencoding. *J. Neuroeng. Rehabil.* **2018**, *15*, 21. [CrossRef] [PubMed]
16. Jiang, N.; Vujaklija, I.; Rehbaum, H.; Graimann, B.; Farina, D. Is Accurate Mapping of EMG Signals on Kinematics Needed for Precise Online Myoelectric Control? *IEEE Trans. Neural Syst. Rehabil. Eng.* **2014**, *22*, 549–558. [CrossRef]
17. Hahne, J.M.; Markovic, M.; Farina, D. User adaptation in Myoelectric Man-Machine Interfaces. *Sci. Rep.* **2017**, *7*, 4437. [CrossRef] [PubMed]

18. Young, A.J.; Hargrove, L.J.; Kuiken, T.A. The Effects of Electrode Size and Orientation on the Sensitivity of Myoelectric Pattern Recognition Systems to Electrode Shift. *IEEE Trans. Biomed. Eng.* **2011**, *58*, 2537–2544. [CrossRef] [PubMed]
19. Abdoli-Eramaki, M.; Damecour, C.; Christenson, J.; Stevenson, J. The Effect of Perspiration on the sEMG Amplitude and Power Spectrum. *J. Electromyography Kinesiol.* **2012**, *22*, 908–913. [CrossRef] [PubMed]
20. Farina, D.; Jiang, N.; Rehbaum, H.; Holobar, A.; Graimann, B.; Dietl, H.; Aszmann, O.C. The extraction of neural information from the surface EMG for the control of upper-limb prostheses: Emerging avenues and challenges. *IEEE Trans. Neural Syst. Rehabil. Eng.* **2014**, *22*, 797–809. [CrossRef] [PubMed]
21. Nishikawa, D.; Yu, W.; Maruishi, M.; Watanabe, I.; Yokoi, H.; Mano, Y.; Kakazu, Y. On-line Learning Based Electromyogram to Forearm Motion Classifier with Motor Skill Evaluation. *JSME Int. J. Ser. C* **2000**, *43*, 906–915. [CrossRef]
22. Kato, R.; Yokoi, H.; Arai, T. Real-time Learning Method for Adaptable Motion-Discrimination using Surface EMG Signal. In Proceedings of the 2006 IEEE/RSJ International Conference on Intelligent Robots and Systems, Beijing, China, 9–15 October 2006; pp. 2127–2132. [CrossRef]
23. Sensinger, J.; Lock, B.; Kuiken, T. Adaptive Pattern Recognition of Myoelectric Signals: Exploration of Conceptual Framework and Practical Algorithms. *IEEE Trans. Neural Syst. Rehabil. Eng.* **2009**, *17*, 270–278. [CrossRef] [PubMed]
24. Chen, X.; Zhang, D.; Zhu, X. Application of a self-enhancing classification method to electromyography pattern recognition for multifunctional prosthesis control. *J. NeuroEng. Rehabil.* **2013**, *10*, 44. [CrossRef]
25. Vidovic, M.M.C.; Hwang, H.J.; Amsuss, S.; Hahne, J.M.; Farina, D.; Muller, K.R. Improving the Robustness of Myoelectric Pattern Recognition for Upper Limb Prostheses by Covariate Shift Adaptation. *IEEE Trans. Neural Syst. Rehabil. Eng.* **2016**, *24*, 961–970. [CrossRef] [PubMed]
26. Zhu, X.; Liu, J.; Zhang, D.; Sheng, X.; Jiang, N. Cascaded Adaptation Framework for Fast Calibration of Myoelectric Control. *IEEE Trans. Neural Syst. Rehabil. Eng.* **2017**, *25*, 254–264. [CrossRef] [PubMed]
27. Prahm, C.; Schulz, A.; Paaben, B.; Schoisswohl, J.; Kaniusas, E.; Dorffner, G.; Hammer, B.; Aszmann, O. Counteracting Electrode Shifts in Upper-Limb Prosthesis Control via Transfer Learning. *IEEE Trans. Neural Syst. Rehabil. Eng.* **2019**, *27*, 956–962. [CrossRef]
28. Gijsberts, A.; Bohra, R.; Sierra González, D.; Werner, A.; Nowak, M.; Caputo, B.; Roa, M.A.; Castellini, C. Stable myoelectric control of a hand prosthesis using non-linear incremental learning. *Front. Neurorobot.* **2014**, *8*, 8. [CrossRef] [PubMed]
29. Hahne, J.M.; Dahne, S.; Hwang, H.J.; Muller, K.R.; Parra, L.C. Concurrent Adaptation of Human and Machine Improves Simultaneous and Proportional Myoelectric Control. *IEEE Trans. Neural Syst. Rehabil. Eng.* **2015**, *23*, 618–627. [CrossRef] [PubMed]
30. Couraud, M.; Cattaert, D.; Paclet, F.; Oudeyer, P.Y.; de Rugy, A. Model and experiments to optimize co-adaptation in a simplified myoelectric control system. *J. Neural Eng.* **2018**, *15*, 026006. [CrossRef] [PubMed]
31. Astrom, K.J.K.J.; Wittenmark, B. *Adaptive Control*; Dover Publications: Mineola, NY, USA, 2008; p. 573.
32. Fortescue, T.; Kershenbaum, L.; Ydstie, B. Implementation of self-tuning regulators with variable forgetting factors. *Automatica* **1981**, *17*, 831–835. [CrossRef]
33. Kulhavý, R.; Kárný, M. Tracking of Slowly Varying Parameters by Directional Forgetting. *IFAC Proc. Vol.* **1984**, *17*, 687–692. [CrossRef]
34. Jiang, N.; Rehbaum, H.; Vujaklija, I.; Graimann, B.; Farina, D. Intuitive, Online, Simultaneous, and Proportional Myoelectric Control Over Two Degrees-of-Freedom in Upper Limb Amputees. *IEEE Trans. Neural Syst. Rehabil. Eng.* **2014**, *22*, 501–510. [CrossRef]
35. Lin, C.; Wang, B.; Jiang, N.; Farina, D. Robust extraction of basis functions for simultaneous and proportional myoelectric control via sparse non-negative matrix factorization. *J. Neural Eng.* **2018**, *15*, 026017. [CrossRef]
36. Rehbaum, H.; Farina, D. Adaptive common average filtering for myocontrol applications. *Med. Biol. Eng. Comput.* **2015**, *53*, 179–186. [CrossRef]
37. Clancy, E.A.; Morin, E.L.; Merletti, R. Sampling, noise-reduction and amplitude estimation issues in surface electromyography. *J. Electromyogr. Kinesiol.* **2002**, *12*, 1–16. [CrossRef]
38. Cao, L.; Schwartz, H. A Directional Forgetting Algorithm Based on the Decomposition of the Information Matrix. *Automatica* **2000**, *36*, 1725–1731. [CrossRef]

39. MacKenzie, I.S. A note on the information-theoretic basis of Fitts' law. *J. Motor Behav.* **1989**, *21*, 323–330. [CrossRef]
40. Brown, M.B.; Forsythe, A.B. Robust Tests for the Equality of Variances. *J. Am. Stat. Assoc.* **1974**, *69*, 364. [CrossRef]

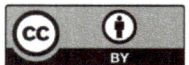

© 2019 by the authors. Licensee MDPI, Basel, Switzerland. This article is an open access article distributed under the terms and conditions of the Creative Commons Attribution (CC BY) license (http://creativecommons.org/licenses/by/4.0/).

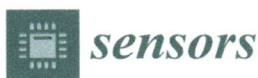

Article

Evaluation of Optimal Vibrotactile Feedback for Force-Controlled Upper Limb Myoelectric Prostheses

Andrea Gonzalez-Rodriguez, Jose L. Ramon, Vicente Morell, Gabriel J. Garcia, Jorge Pomares, Carlos A. Jara and Andres Ubeda *

Human Robotics Group, University of Alicante, 03690 Alicante, Spain; aerdna.gr@gmail.com (A.G.-R.); jl.ramon@ua.es (J.L.R.); vicente.morell@ua.es (V.M.); gjgg@ua.es (G.J.G.); jpomares@ua.es (J.P.); carlos.jara@ua.es (C.A.J.)
* Correspondence: andres.ubeda@ua.es; Tel.: +34-965-903-400 (ext. 1094)

Received: 30 September 2019; Accepted: 26 November 2019; Published: 28 November 2019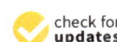

Abstract: The main goal of this study is to evaluate how to optimally select the best vibrotactile pattern to be used in a closed loop control of upper limb myoelectric prostheses as a feedback of the exerted force. To that end, we assessed both the selection of actuation patterns and the effects of the selection of frequency and amplitude parameters to discriminate between different feedback levels. A single vibrotactile actuator has been used to deliver the vibrations to subjects participating in the experiments. The results show no difference between pattern shapes in terms of feedback perception. Similarly, changes in amplitude level do not reflect significant improvement compared to changes in frequency. However, decreasing the number of feedback levels increases the accuracy of feedback perception and subject-specific variations are high for particular participants, showing that a fine-tuning of the parameters is necessary in a real-time application to upper limb prosthetics. In future works, the effects of training, location, and number of actuators will be assessed. This optimized selection will be tested in a real-time proportional myocontrol of a prosthetic hand.

Keywords: vibrotactile actuation; sensory feedback; prosthetics

---

1. Introduction

An amputation is the removal of a limb caused by a trauma, a medical condition, or surgery. Negative impacts to the amputee include the loss of function and sensory perception of the limb as well as changes in their interaction with the environment that may lead to psychological conditions. Limb prosthetics are used to limit the effects of this trauma. A prosthesis can be defined as an artificial replacement of the lost limb to regain independence after the amputation. Active prostheses allow the user to interact with their environment, e.g., by opening and closing an artificial hand to grasp objects [1]. One of the most common control methods is the use of the residual electrical activity of the nerves measured on the stump as an input to the prosthesis. This kind of control is called myoelectric and it naturally replicates how healthy individuals control their limbs [2].

One of the main issues of upper limb myoelectric prostheses is the way of dealing with sensory feedback [3]. Open-loop prostheses only account for visual feedback of how the grasping is achieved, so users do not have precise information of grasping forces leading to difficulties in the manipulation of fragile objects. Indeed, most current commercial prostheses only provide feedforward control of grasping. To solve this problem, precise sensors can be used in the prosthetic hand to give back force information to the user during its operation [4,5]. The closed-loop approach can then be achieved in several ways. One way is to provide meaningful visual feedback of the exerted force. e.g., by adding visual force information on the prosthetic hand [6]. One way of addressing this approach is the use of virtual environments delivering information of a simulated upper limb [7]. The use of visual feedback of the actual neuromuscular processes that are taking place has emerged as an effective way to increase user involvement [8]. In a recent study, a novel visual feedback approach is proposed as a combination of force information with electromyographic biofeedback to enhance sensory perception [9]. Auditory feedback has been also applied alone or in combination with visual feedback [10].

Other methods are based on providing actual physical sensations to the user. Vibrotactile feedback is the most used method to provide force information during grasping tasks [11–14]. Vibrotactile actuators are lightweight and small and deliver tactile feedback through vibration patterns. Vibrotactile actuation can provide additional sensory information in a broad number of domains ranging from leisure activities to rehabilitation performance [15,16]. Designing an effective vibrotactile feedback system allows users to perceive and respond to force stimuli correctly. In the field of rehabilitation, vibrotactile feedback is commonly used for both upper and lower limb prostheses [17,18]. Another similar approach is the use of mechanotactile actuation [19]. In contrast to vibrotactile feedback, this technology has a better resolution, making it easier to distinguish between different force levels, but it is heavier and larger. Force feedback can also be delivered through electrical stimulation [20,21]. However, this method can be painful and unpleasant to the user if the signal amplitude is too large. This is especially critical if stimulation is performed invasively [22].

Besides the effective introduction of force feedback in current commercial prostheses, one major aspect that still needs to be properly assessed is how well these previously described methods can discriminate between different force levels, i.e., given the method, how to provide the user with a robust, reliable and easy to embody force feedback approach. To date, several studies have dealt with the comparison of different types of feedback added to the control scheme [23]. This concept is generally defined as multisensory feedback [24]. However, little attention has been paid to a precise parameter tuning in the delivered patterns.

For the lower limb, a few studies have focused on determining how to select certain parameters of the vibrotactile feedback. For instance, aspects such as number of actuators and location, delivered frequencies or habituation to the stimulus have been assessed [25,26]. In general, studies on vibrotactile feedback use no more than five different feedback levels [27] and do not focus specifically on the type of stimulus pattern that is delivered. This is also common in other feedback approaches.

The main goal of this study is to evaluate the latter aspect in a well-established method such as vibrotactile actuation. To that end, we have assessed both the selection of actuation patterns and the effects of the selection of frequency and amplitude parameters to discriminate between different feedback levels that could be then assigned to different levels of the exerted force of the prosthesis. The experimental protocol is proposed as a tool for optimally selecting the best vibrotactile pattern to be used in a closed loop control of upper limb myoelectric prostheses.

2. Materials and Methods

Nine subjects participated in the study (6 male and 3 female aged 26.4 ± 3.2 years old). All subjects were in perfect physical condition with no history of neurological disease. The experimental setup was very simple. Vibrations were delivered with different parameters to study the optimal vibrotactile pattern. The FeelVibe actuator (I-CubeX, Infusion Systems) is based on an Eccentric Rotating Mass (ERM) motor with a haptic driver. The actuator dimensions are $19 \times 19 \times 7$ mm, making it ideal for placement in adequate positions of the amputated limb, either the arm or the stump itself. In the present study the actuator was placed on the forearm of the participants (see Figure 1) .

The FeelVibe actuator is connected to a digitizer WiDig with up to 8-channel capability, allowing for multiple vibrating sources. This digitizer is connected through USB to the computer and actuated using Touch Sense 2200 software with a VirtualMIDI driver, which allows delivering up to 123 predefined vibration patterns. From this set of patterns, different combinations have been selected to configure the experimental protocol.

Two different sets of vibrations were applied:

- **Pattern shape:** For this set, subjects were provided with vibrotactile feedback of different patterns. Feedback levels were simulated by increasing and decreasing the time lag (tp) between three consecutive vibration peaks. The vibrating frequency of the onset segments was fixed by the hardware and was felt by subjects as a continuous stimulus. The time lag was selected in a scale between 0.1 to 1 s in steps of 0.1 s, making a total of 10 different feedback levels. A maximum tp of 1 s was selected to avoid long response times in a future application of these patterns to a real-time prosthetic control. A total of 5 different patterns (see Figure 2) were evaluated. Each feedback level was repeated 5 times and randomly delivered to the subject making a total of 100 trials per pattern.
- **Pattern amplitude:** For this set, Pattern 3 was selected and amplitude was changed between 20% to 100% in steps of 20% making a total of 5 feedback levels. This pattern was selected as it was the only predefined pattern that could provide different amplitude levels. The number of feedback levels was limited to 5 due to the amplitude resolution provided by the device. Each feedback level was repeated 10 times and randomly delivered to the subject making a total of 50 trials.

Before starting the experiments, subjects were asked if they were capable of feeling differences between all consecutive feedback levels. We checked this with all subjects and all answered positive. Subjects were then asked to evaluate the patterns using two possible approaches: relative difference and absolute level. For the first one, subjects were asked to say if the current pattern was softer, stronger, or equal compared to the previous by voting $+1$, -1, or 0, respectively. The first vibration was not voted and served as reference for the remaining. In a second run, subjects were provided again with the same set of vibrations and were asked to determine the exact feedback level by voting from 1 to 10.

To record subject replies and easily deliver the selected patterns, a customized Matlab software has been implemented. This software communicates with WiDig digitizer through the serial port and allows saving all the experimental information in an *xls* file for future analysis.

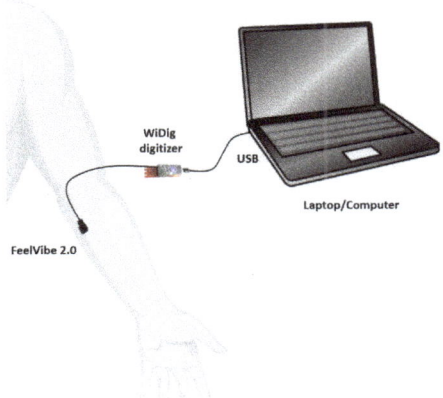

Figure 1. Experimental set-up.

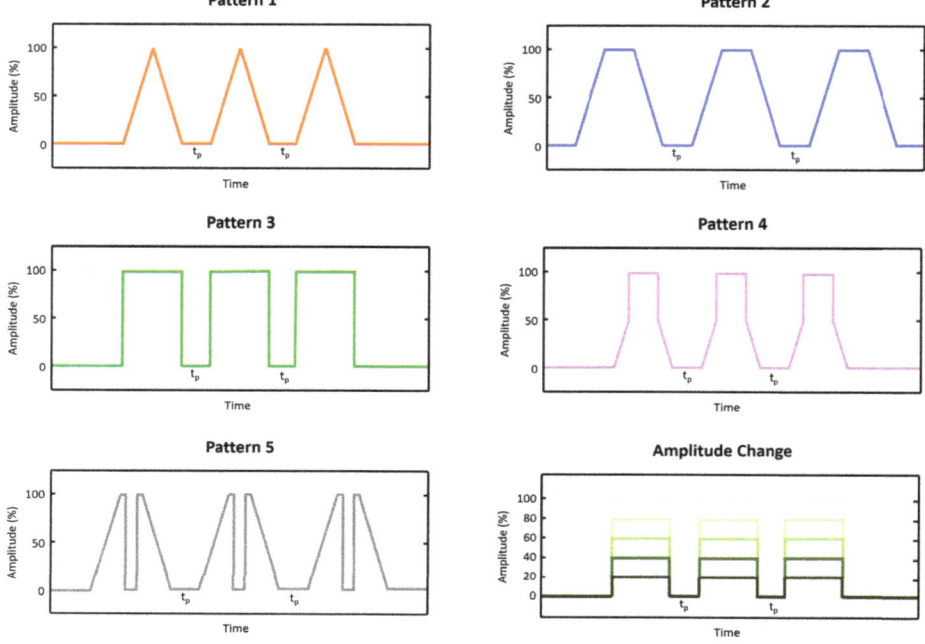

Figure 2. Vibration patterns delivered to the subjects.

3. Results

Figure 3 shows the success rate obtained for different patterns when taking into account relative difference between consecutive stimulations. Results are similar for most of the subjects, with an average of 75.7% ± 0.9% (Figure 3, left). Only subject 8 (63.4% ± 4.9%) and subject 4 (43.2% ± 2.1%) are significantly lower (Wilcoxon Signed-Rank Test, $p < 0.05$ with a Bonferroni–Holm correction). The worst performance of these subjects is stable for all the evaluated patterns. The average results per pattern indicate that all of them are similarly distinguished in their variation (Figure 3, right). Interestingly, changes in pattern frequency and changes in amplitude do not show significant differences in performance (Wilcoxon Signed-Rank Test, $p > 0.05$ with a Bonferroni–Holm correction). In Figure 4, success rates for an exact match of the feedback level are shown. The results show that subjects have a low accuracy in their perception of absolute values with an average of 32.6% ± 4.0% (Figure 4, top-left). This means that subjects can accurately perceive only around one third of the delivered feedback levels. As in the previous analysis, differences across subjects are not very high. Subjects 4 and 9 are again the lowest, with rates of 24.8% ± 9.7% and 21.2% ± 8.1%, respectively. However, these differences are, in this case, nonsignificant (Wilcoxon Signed-Rank Test, $p > 0.05$ with a Bonferroni–Holm correction). As for the previous approach, patterns 1 to 5 do not show significant differences (Wilcoxon Signed-Rank Test, $p > 0.05$ with a Bonferroni–Holm correction). Note that, in contrast to the relative difference approach, where intrasubject success rate was very stable, the standard deviation increases to ~10%, meaning that certain patterns are more difficult to be perceived by subjects. An illustrative example of this is Subject 4, who achieves very low accuracy for Pattern 1: an 8% compared to the remaining patterns where more than 20% accuracy is obtained.

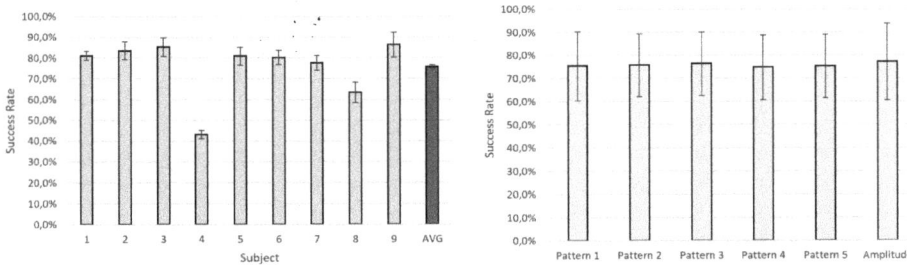

Figure 3. Average success rate (%) in the evaluation of the relative differences of pattern shapes (1 to 5) and pattern amplitude. Results per subject (**left**). Results per pattern (**right**).

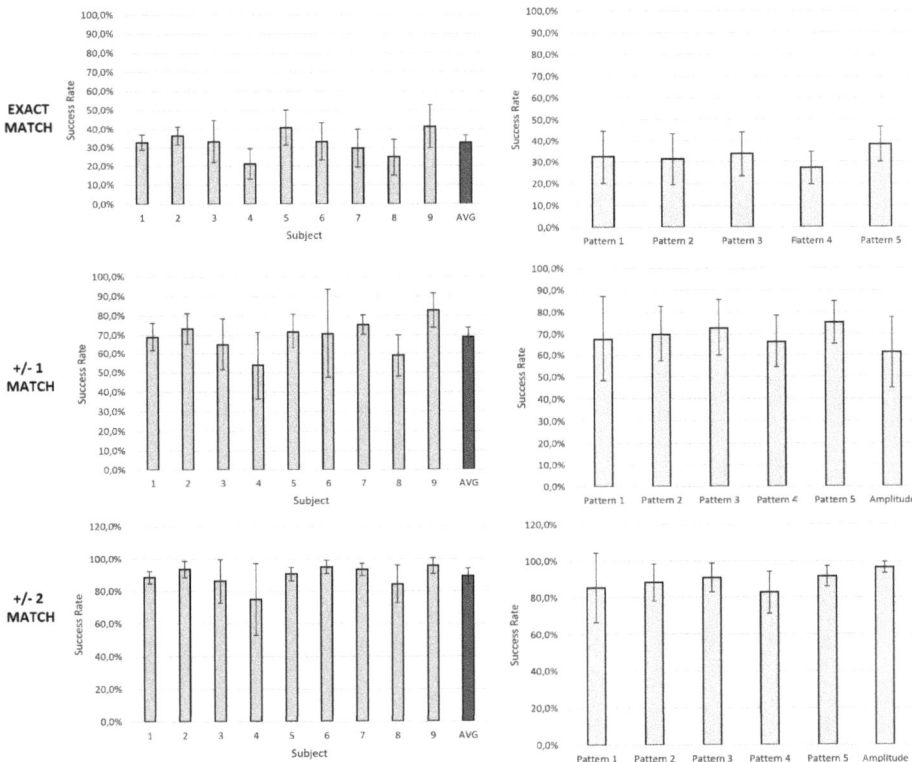

Figure 4. Average success rate (%) in the evaluation of the absolute feedback values for pattern shapes (1 to 5) and pattern amplitude. The first row represents exact matches in feedback level perception. The second row represents close matches (no further than 1 in error) in feedback perception. The third row represents further matches (no further than 2 in error) in feedback perception. Amplitude change success rate is only showed for the second and third row.

To evaluate the convenience of using amplitude changes instead of frequency variation of the vibrotactile patterns, absolute matches have been computed again with a maximum error of one level only for patterns 1 to 5 (frequency change). This allows evaluating success rate of only 5 different levels to be compared to the 5 different amplitude levels delivered in the second set of vibrations.

As expected, success rate increases to an average of ~69.0% ± 5.0% (Figure 4, bottom-left). This is very similar for all 5 patterns (Figure 4, bottom-right). However, success rate in feedback amplitude changes is slightly lower (61.4% ± 16.5%) but again they do not show significant differences (Wilcoxon Signed-Rank Test, $p > 0.05$ with a Bonferroni–Holm correction). An additional comparison has been made by increasing the possibility of error in perception to a maximum error of two. In that case, success rate increases to almost 100%. Differences between subjects and approaches continue to be nonsignificant but intrasubject accuracy across patterns is the same or even increases with very high deviations for particular subjects (4 and 8).

For the last analysis, the correlation between perceived and delivered feedback has been evaluated by showing how well subjects selected the correct delivered feedback level in average (Figure 5). For all patterns, there is a high correlation 0.92% ± 0.04%. Patterns 1 to 5 show correlations above 0.9. However, amplitude changes are not so well correlated (0.82). From the graph, it can be clearly seen that high feedback levels are generally perceived as a lower feedback level. Another interesting aspect is that with a higher resolution in delivered feedback levels (patterns 1 to 5), subjects have more difficulties to perceive differences. In Figure 5, only the amplitude change curve (with only 5 levels) is increasing monotonically.

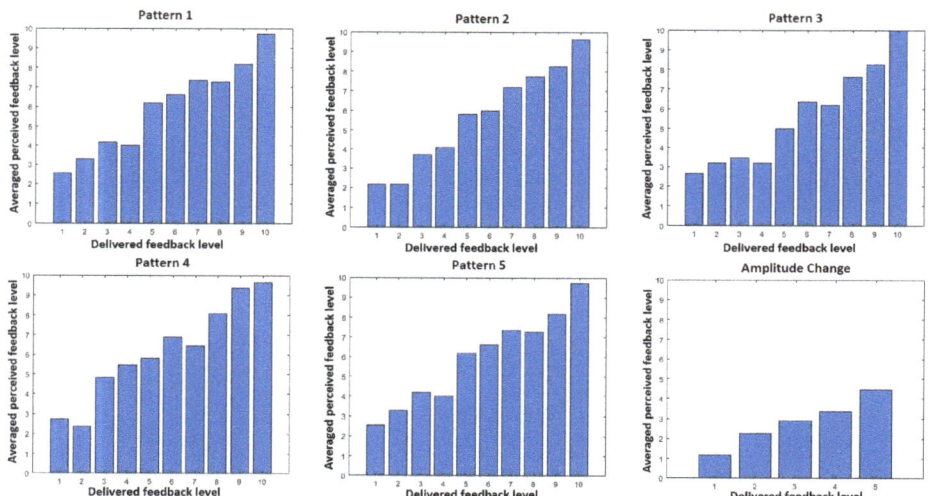

Figure 5. Correlation between perceived and delivered feedback levels for all 6 patterns.

4. Discussion

One of the primary goals of this study was to select the best vibrotactile pattern to be used as feedback for the force control of an upper limb prostheses. To this end, different pattern shapes were evaluated discriminating feedback levels that corresponded to force levels. Stimulation trains were delivered to the subjects by varying the vibration frequency. The results show that the pattern shape has a small influence in the feedback level perception and there is no significant difference between the selected patterns (Figures 3 and 4). Therefore, when tuning parameters of vibrotactile feedback, other factors need to be considered. In this study, we assume two different perspectives—frequency tuning or amplitude tuning—and, in this case, the frequency tuning approach led to a slightly better perception of feedback levels but nonsignificant. Previous studies show that high frequencies are better perceived than low frequencies [26], this may be the result of the fact that the amplitude and the frequency are coupled for ERM motors. One possible reason why these differences are not appreciated in our study is that changes in frequency of delivered trains reached a maximum of ~10 Hz and were much smaller that in [26], so the effect of the coupling was not present. Although further experiments must be done to evaluate this differences, the results suggest that in a real-tune application of vibrotactile feedback, delivered feedback levels are similarly perceived in terms of vibration frequency and amplitude level.

Another key factor is how many feedback levels are subjects capable of differentiating with enough accuracy. Figure 4 indicates that 10 different feedback levels are difficult to perceive (32.6% ± 4.0%). When this number of feedback levels is decreased to five, the success rate importantly increases (69.0% ± 5.0%), and it is even higher when up to two levels perception error is allowed (89.2% ± 4.9%). Determining the optimal number of levels to discriminate depends on the subject perception capabilities and the approach used to deliver difference in feedback levels (frequency or amplitude). A fine-tuning of these parameters is necessary to optimally apply this kind of sensory feedback. In fact, most of the current studies do not include more than five different feedback levels [27]. Proportional myoelectric control, in which a non-finite feedback level is needed, may benefit from a correct selection of the number of delivered feedback levels. Decrease in feedback perception was present for subjects 4 and 9. In those cases, subjects had more difficulties in discriminating feedback levels. This suggests that sensorimotor perception is very subject-dependent. Indeed, many patterns differ significantly for particular subjects that show a very high standard deviation. A possible way of reducing this perception error may come through a proper training protocol.

Our study is limited to a particular set of vibration patterns and tuning parameters. In future works, we will analyze effects of training or habituation, location, and number of actuators. Additionally, a comparison of different frequency and amplitude resolutions, i.e., number of perceived feedback levels, will be performed to define the maximum number of feedback levels that can be optimally distinguished. As previously mentioned, these aspects have already been partially addressed in other studies for the lower-limb [25,26], but a systematic evaluation on the upper limb is necessary as a big number of prosthetic devices are used by transradial amputees. Location and number of actuators can be explored to evaluate effects in perception error, for instance, by adding additional vibration trains in different body parts or changing their location to a more sensitive area. An interesting approach to this issue has been evaluated in [25], where an array of multiple actuators is places from the proximal to the distal part of the thigh. Others factors not included in previous studies are the effects of a continuous feedback versus a discrete one and the suitability of the proposed patterns in terms of subject time response, which is a critical factor in closed loop control. To evaluate the tuning of vibrotactile parameters, real-time proportional myocontrol of a prosthetic hand will be combined with vibrotactile sensory feedback. Vibrotactile patterns will be delivered proportional to the exerted force of the robotic hand measured from force sensors. This will help to determine how well a properly tuned feedback increases grasping accuracy and force perception. In this context, factors such as the influence of the socket in the perception of the vibration patterns can as well be examined.

Author Contributions: Definition of experiments, A.G.-R. and A.U.; experimentation, validation, and formal analysis, A.G.-R.; manuscript writing, A.G.-R. and A.U.; review and edition of the manuscript, J.L.R., V.M., G.J.G., J.P., C.A.J., and A.U.; supervision, C.A.J. and A.U.

Funding: This research was funded by University of Alicante through project "Control Platform for a Robotic Hand based on Electromyographic Signals" (GRE16-20).

Conflicts of Interest: The authors declare no conflicts of interest.

References

1. Ribeiro, J.; Mota, F.; Cavalcante, T.; Nogueira, I.; Gondim, V.; Albuquerque, V.; Alexandria, A. Analysis of man-machine interfaces in upper limb prosthesis: A review. *Robotics* **2019**, *8*, 16. [CrossRef]
2. Geethanjali, P. Myoelectric control of prosthetic hands: State-of-the-art review. *Med. Devices* **2016**, *9*, 247–255. [CrossRef] [PubMed]
3. Antfolk, C.; D'Alonzo, M.; Rosén, B.; Lundborg, G.; Sebelius, F.; Cipriani, C. Sensory feedback in upper limb prosthetics. *Expert Rev. Med. Devices* **2013**, *10*, 45–54. [CrossRef] [PubMed]

4. Ciancio, A.L.; Cordella, F.; Barone, R.; Romeo, R.A.; Bellingegni, A.D.; Sacchetti, R.; Davalli, A.; Di Pino, G.; Ranieri, F.; Di Lazzaro, V.; et al. Control of Prosthetic Hands via the Peripheral Nervous System. *Front. Neurosci.* **2016**, *10*, 116. [CrossRef]
5. Trujillo, M.S.; Russell, D.M.; Anderson, D.I.; Mitchell, M. Grip Force Control Using Prosthetic and Anatomical Limbs. *J. Prosthetics Orthot.* **2014**, *30*, 132–139. [CrossRef]
6. Engeberg, D.E.; Meek, M. Enhanced visual feedback for slip prevention with a prosthetic hand. *Prosthetics Orthot. Int.* **2012**, *36*, 423–429. [CrossRef] [PubMed]
7. Clemente, F.; Dosen, S.; Lonini, L.; Markovic, M.; Farina, D.; Cipriani, C. Humans can integrate augmented reality feedback in their sensorimotor control of a robotic hand. *IEEE Trans. Human-Mach. Syst.* **2017**, *47*, 583–589. [CrossRef]
8. Giggins, O.M.; McCarthy, U.; Caulfield, B. Biofeedback in rehabilitation. *J. Neuroeng. Rehabil.* **2013**, *10*, 60. [CrossRef]
9. Došen, S.; Markovic, M.; Somer, K.; Graimann, B.; Farina, D. EMG Biofeedback for online predictive control of grasping force in a myoelectric prosthesis. *J. Neuroeng. Rehabil.* **2015**, *12*, 55. [CrossRef]
10. Shehata, A.W.; Scheme, E.J.; Sensinger, J.W. Audible Feedback Improves Internal Model Strength and Performance of Myoelectric Prosthesis Control. *Nat. Sci. Rep.* **2018**, *8*, 8541. [CrossRef]
11. Markovic, M.; Schweisfurth, M.A.; Engels, L.; Bentz, T.; Wüstefeld, D.; Farina, D.; Dosen, S. The clinical relevance of advanced artificial feedback in the control of a multi-functional myoelectric prosthesis. *J. Neuroeng. Rehabil.* **2018**, *15*, 28. [CrossRef] [PubMed]
12. Pena, A.E.; Rincon-Gonzalez, L.; Abbas, J.J.; Jung, R. Effects of vibrotactile feedback and grasp interface compliance on perception and control of a sensorized myoelectric hand. *PLoS ONE* **2019**, *14*, e0210956. [CrossRef] [PubMed]
13. Raveh, E.; Friedman, J.; Portnoy, S. Evaluation of the effects of adding vibrotactile feedback to myoelectric prosthesis users on performance and visual attention in a dual-task paradigm. *Clin. Rehabil.* **2018**, *32*, 1308–1316. [CrossRef] [PubMed]
14. Witteveen, H.J.; Rietman, H.S.; Veltink, P.H. Vibrotactile grasping force and hand aperture feedback for myoelectric forearm prosthesis users. *Prosthetics Orthot. Int.* **2015**, *39*, 204–212. [CrossRef]
15. Held, J.P.; Klaassen, B.; van Beijnum, B.-J.F.; Luft, A.R.; Veltink, P.H. Usability evaluation of a vibrotactile feedback system in stroke subjects. *Front. Bioeng. Biotechnol.* **2017**, *4*, 98. [CrossRef]
16. Li, Y.; Jeon, W.R.; Nam, C.S. Navigation by vibration: Effects of vibrotactile feedback on a navigation task. *Int. J. Ind. Ergon.* **2015**, *46*, 76–84. [CrossRef]
17. Guemann, M.; Bouvier, S.; Halgand, C.; Borrini, L.; Paclet, F.; Lapeyre, E.; Ricard, D.; Cattaert, D.; de Rugy, A. Sensory and motor parameter estimation for elbow myoelectric control with vibrotactile feedback. *Ann. Phys. Rehabil. Med.* **2018**, *61*, e467. [CrossRef]
18. Thomas, N.; Ung, G.; McGarvey, C.; Brown, J.D. Comparison of vibrotactile and joint-torque feedback in a myoelectric upper limb prosthesis. *J. Neuroeng. Rehabil.* **2019**, *16*, 70. [CrossRef]
19. Antfolk, C.; D'Alonzo, M.; Controzzi, M.; Lundborg, G.; Rosén, B.; Sebelius, F.; Cipriani, C. Artificial redirection of sensation from prosthetic fingers to the phantom hand map on transradial amputees: Vibrotactile versus mechanotactile sensory feedback. *IEEE Trans. Neural Syst. Rehabil. Eng.* **2013**, *21*, 112–120. [CrossRef]
20. Isaković, M.; Belić, M.; Štrbac, M.; Popović, D.; Došen, S.; Farina, D.; Keller, T. Electrotactile feedback improves performance and facilitates learning in the routine grasping task. *Eur. J. Transl. Myol.* **2016**, *26*, 6069. [CrossRef]
21. Schweisfurth, M.; Markovic, M.; Dosen, S.; Teich, F.; Graimann, B.; Farina, D. Electrotactile EMG feedback improves the control of prosthesis grasping force. *J. Neural Eng.* **2016**, *13*, 056010. [CrossRef] [PubMed]
22. Schiefer, M.; Tan, D.; Sidek, S.M.; Tyler, D.J. Sensory feedback by peripheral nerve stimulation improves task performance in individuals with upper limb loss using a myoelectric prosthesis. *J. Neural Eng.* **2016**, *13*, 016001. [CrossRef] [PubMed]
23. Engels, L.F.; Shehata, A.W.; Scheme, E.J.; Sensinger, J.W.; Cipriani, C. When less is more—Discrete tactile feedback dominates continuous audio biofeedback in the integrated percept while controlling a myoelectric prosthetic hand. *Front. Neurosci.* **2019**, *13*, 578. [CrossRef] [PubMed]
24. Rognini, G.; Petrini, F.M.; Raspopovic, S.; Valle, G.; Granata, G.; Strauss, I.; Solcà, M.; Bello-Ruiz, J.; Herbelin, B.; Mange, R.; et al. Multisensory bionic limb to achieve prosthesis embodiment and reduce distorted phantom limb perceptions. *J. Neurol. Neurosurg. Psychiatry* **2018**, *90*, 833–836. [CrossRef]

25. Sharma, A.; Torres-Moreno, R.; Zabjek, K; Andrysek, J. Toward an artificial sensory feedback system for prosthetic mobility rehabilitation: Examination of sensorimotor responses. *J. Rehabil. Res. Dev.* **2014** *51*, 907–918. [CrossRef]
26. Wentink, E.C.; Mulder, A.; Rietman, J.S.; Veltink, P.H. Vibrotactile stimulation of the upper leg: Effects of location, stimulation method and habituation. In Proceedings of the 33rd Annual International Conference of the IEEE EMBS, Boston, MA, USA, 30 August–3 September 2011; pp. 1668–1671.
27. Stephens-Fripp, B.; Alici, G.; Mutlu, R. A Review of Non-Invasive Sensory Feedback Methods for Transradial Prosthetic Hands. *IEEE Access* **2018**, *6*, 6878–6899. [CrossRef]

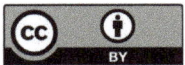

© 2019 by the authors. Licensee MDPI, Basel, Switzerland. This article is an open access article distributed under the terms and conditions of the Creative Commons Attribution (CC BY) license (http://creativecommons.org/licenses/by/4.0/).

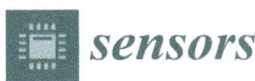

Article

HYBRID: Ambulatory Robotic Gait Trainer with Movement Induction and Partial Weight Support

Eloy Urendes [1,†,*], Guillermo Asín-Prieto [2], Ramón Ceres [1], Rodrigo García-Carmona [1], Rafael Raya [1] and José L. Pons [2,3,4,5]

1. Department of Information Systems Engineering, University San Pablo CEU, Boadilla del Monte, 28688 Madrid, Spain; ramon.ceresruiz@colaborador.ceu.es (R.C.); rodrigo.garciacarmona@ceu.es (R.G.-C.); rafael.rayalopez@ceu.es (R.R.)
2. Neural Rehabilitation Group, Cajal Institute, CSIC—Spanish National Research Council, 28002 Madrid, Spain; guillermo.asin.prieto@csic.es (G.A.-P.); jpons@sralab.org (J.L.P.)
3. Legs & Walking AbilityLab, Shirley Ryan AbilityLab, Chicago, IL 60611, USA
4. Department Biomedical Engineering & Department Mechanical Engineering, McCormick School of Engineering, Northwestern University, Evanston, IL 60208, USA
5. Department of PM&R, Feinberg School of Medicine, Northwestern University, Chicago, IL 60611, USA
* Correspondence: eloyjose.urendesjimenez@ceu.es; Tel.: +34-91-372-47-00 (ext. 14963)
† Current address: Eloy Urendes, Escuela Politecnica Superior, Universidad San Pablo CEU, Urb. Monteprincipe S/N, Boadilla del Monte, 28668 Madrid, Spain.

Received: 30 September 2019; Accepted: 31 October 2019; Published: 2 November 2019

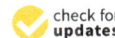

Abstract: Robotic exoskeletons that induce leg movement have proven effective for lower body rehabilitation, but current solutions offer limited gait patterns, lack stabilization, and do not properly stimulate the proprioceptive and balance systems (since the patient remains in place). Partial body weight support (PBWS) systems unload part of the patient's body weight during rehabilitation, improving the locomotive capabilities and minimizing the muscular effort. HYBRID is a complete system that combines a 6DoF lower body exoskeleton (H1) with a PBWS system (REMOVI) to produce a solution apt for clinical practice that offers improves on existing devices, moves with the patient, offers a gait cycle extracted from the kinematic analysis of healthy users, records the session data, and can easily transfer the patient from a wheelchair to standing position. This system was developed with input from therapists, and its response times have been measured to ensure it works swiftly and without a perceptible delay.

Keywords: gait; trainer; partial weight suspension; induction of movements; disability; exoskeleton; lower body rehabilitation; robotic rehabilitation

1. Introduction

Assisted gait training and rehabilitation have a high impact on healthcare and are characterized by scientific and technical challenges [1–3]. Recent research in this field has translated into several devices, ranging from prostheses and orthoses to walkers and gait trainers, that provide users with aids designed to help with particular disabilities.

There is no consensus on which program is best suited for gait rehabilitation or which tools are most useful, especially for spinal cord injury (SCI) [4,5]. However, repetitive movement strategies have proliferated in clinical practice [6,7]. They are designed to stimulate the central pattern generators (CPGs), responsible for generating coordinated movements [5,8]. This manual-therapy-based training is held back by lack of personnel and the physical effort it demands from the therapist, severely limiting its applicability. Robotics-based rehabilitation offers a unique opportunity to solve this problem, improving training intensity and quality. By assisting both the therapists and the patients in performing a rhythmic and synchronized lower body movement, robotic devices have the potential to greatly reduce the physical effort needed, and thus decrease the injuries of therapists derived from this effort.

2. Related Work

Wearable exoskeletons that can induce musculoskeletal movement, and therefore help the user perform a healthy gait pattern, are a very popular way of using robotic devices for rehabilitation. Most of them, like Ekso Bionics [9], HAL [10], Vanderbilt exoskeleton [11], or ReWalk [12] are 4DoF (degrees of freedom) lower-limb exoskeletons, and actuate both the hip and knee on the sagittal plane. Recent studies [13,14] have demonstrated that training using HAL is effective in improving ambulatory mobility for patients with stroke or spinal cord injury. Robotic training led to an improvement in walking parameters and in balance abilities, with increases in the WISCI-II score. Similar results have been achieved using Ekso Bionics [15]. Other devices such as MindWalker [16], CUHK-EXO [17], or XoR2 [18] include hip rotation. These ambulatory exoskeletons need crutches to provide stabilization and control the lateral balance during movement. This setup is infeasible for patients that lack good upper body strength or biomechanical coordination. On top of that, they introduce the risk of falls and produce fatigue. These factors make such exoskeletons impractical for many users.

This problem could be avoided by using PBWS (partial body weight support) solutions that unload part of the patient's body weight by suspending them. This way, the percentage of body weight that the lower body must support during rehabilitation therapy can be tightly controlled. Such strategies have the potential to improve the locomotive capabilities of people with motor deficit by minimizing the muscular effort required and simultaneously reducing the forces and pressures exerted over the user's skeletal system [19]. Several studies have proved the huge benefits that PBWS solutions have on clinical practice [20,21].

However, PBWS was traditionally implemented using fixed structures with either treadmill or rigid frames. Recent solutions have seen the introduction of robotic gait trainers that can combine assisted leg movement with partial weight suspension. This way, crutches are not needed and falls can be totally avoided. These two features are considered mandatory for patients with systemic motor deficit.

Devices like Lokomat [22], GaitTrainer [23] LOPES [24], ALEX [25] or C-ALEX [26] integrate an exoskeleton for particular body regions with treadmill and PBWS systems. These solutions enable reproducible and intense therapy sessions while logging objective measures to assess the exercise's results. These devices are limited in the sense that the patient remains in place, and therefore their proprioception, posture, and dynamic balance systems are not being properly trained and receive conflicting stimuli.

To address these shortcomings, new ambulatory training systems which allow a higher freedom of movement from the patient have been designed, such as WalkTrainer [27] Nature-gaits [28], SUBAR [29], EXPOS [30], the device presented in [31], MLLRE [32], or MOPASS [33]. However, solutions such as these present several drawbacks, like the inability to easily move the patients from their wheelchairs to standing position. On top of that, these trainers cannot generate a gait movement synchronized with the system's absolute speed or force the patient to maintain a posture conductive to put on an exoskeleton—a process involving important physical effort and lengthy preparation times.

This work tries to bridge this gap by presenting an innovative self-propelled ambulatory system for gait rehabilitation with lower body movement induction, PBWS and body stabilization designed for clinical environments, named HYBRID (Hybrid Technological Platform for Rehabilitation, Functional Compensation and Training of Gait in SCI Patients). Our solution enables practitioners to easily transfer patients from a wheelchair to standing position, suspend their weight, and provide assisted gait patterns extracted from healthy users, all while offering safety and comfort. This system is easy to use for both users and practitioners.

The developed system has been financed by the Spanish *Plan Nacional*, with support from interested partners like the *Hospital Nacional de Parapléjicos de Toledo* (HNPT) and the *Instituto Nacional de Educación Física* (INEF), and has received input from other experts in the fields of rehabilitation and gait analysis, helping to focus on the more relevant design issues.

3. Materials and Methods

The HYBRID device is a gait trainer based on a double support system (Figure 1): a bilateral 3DoF per leg (6DoF total) lower-limb exoskeleton (H1 [34–36]) and a PBWS system (REMOVI). The former is an exoskeleton that can perform a prerecorded walking pattern while registering the angular positions of its six actuated joints (ankles, knees, and hips). The latter is an active PBWS system that supports both the exoskeleton and the user through a harness. For the sake of clarity, this section is divided in three parts, with each of the first two devoted to a different subsystem of HYBRID: H1 and REMOVI. Each part is further divided into several smaller subsections that detail the mechanical structure and electromechanical elements, sensors, and software platform of the H1 and REMOVI modules. Finally, the last part details how the communication between the exoskeleton, the PBWS, and the therapist's computer is achieved.

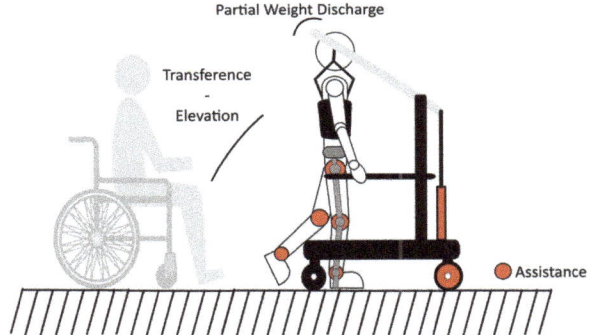

Figure 1. General view of the HYBRID device.

The H1 lower-limb robotic exoskeleton was created by the Neural Rehabilitation Group (NRG) from the Cajal Institute of CSIC as part of the HYPER project [37]. It is built upon the experience acquired in previous projects [38–41] and is under active development [42,43]. The H1 is a medical device designed for the clinical environment, to provide training and rehabilitation of gait over ground for patients suffering from several pathologies, such as stroke, spinal cord injury, or cerebral palsy. It can support cadences of up to 0.5 m/s (1.8 km/h) and produce a gait pattern extracted from the kinematic analysis of healthy users. This exoskeleton can also be locked in a forced standing position, stabilizing the patient by blocking the motors.

The REMOVI PBWS system is a new development designed to reduce the physical effort required by both the patient and the practitioner to a minimum. Toward this aim, it needs to be self-propelled, provide a transfer operation that can move the patient from a wheelchair to standing position (and vice-versa), allow the user to freely walk around with partial weight suspension, and interface and integrate with the H1 exoskeleton module.

3.1. H1 Exoskeleton

3.1.1. Mechanical Structure and Electromechanical Elements

Since gait happens mainly in the sagittal plane, the exoskeleton has been designed to actuate over it. Unlike most exoskeletons (commercially available or in the literature), it also has powered ankles.

This feature is especially important since the ankle bears high torques during gait [44], is responsible for providing balance and attaining the standing position [45,46], and supports considerable body weight [46]. Additionally, heel contact, toe off, and plantar sensitivity play a very important role in balance proprioception [47], and a proper ankle movement is needed to produce these sensations.

The H1 exoskeleton is comprised of two (one per leg) mechanically independent 3DoF lower-limb orthoses, actuated at the hip, knee, and ankle joints in the sagittal plane. Figure 2 shows that each orthosis is made up of four rigid telescopic bars that correspond to the pelvis, femur, tibia, and foot. They are connected by actuation modules (see Figure 3) that match the location of human joints. Both orthoses are connected through a rigid hip structure and a deformable pelvic module made out of polymer, to better adapt to the user's waist and abdominal contour. This setup allows for small adduction and abduction non-actuated hip movements. The exoskeleton is adjustable in width, depth, and height to match the user's characteristics (1.50 m to 1.90 m height, up to 100 kg weight), covering more than 95% of the target population [48].

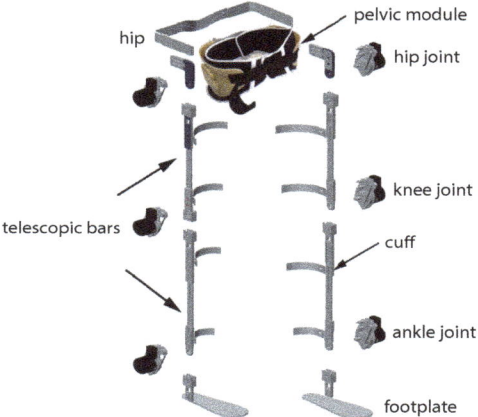

Figure 2. Exploded view of the H1 exoskeleton mechanical structure.

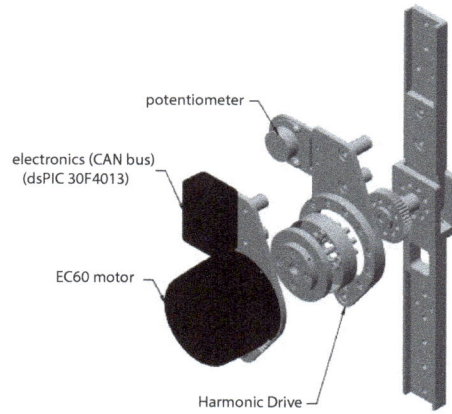

Figure 3. Exploded view of a joint actuation module. CAN: Controller Area Network.

The exoskeleton's range of motion (ROM) corresponds to that of a healthy individual [49] and can be seen in Table 1. This ROM allows users to also perform sit-to-stand and stand-to-sit motions. The H1 design and materials selection has taken into account ergonomics and comfort issues.

Table 1. Actuated degrees of freedom (DoF) and range of motion (ROM) of H1 exoskeleton joints. Sign criteria: positive for flexion (dorsiflexion for ankle) and negative for extension (plantarflexion for ankle).

Joint	DOF	Design	ROM
Hip	Flexo/extension	Actuated	$100°/-20°$
Hip	Addu/abduction	Free	$10°/-10°$
Knee	Flexo/extension	Actuated	$100°/-5°$
Ankle	Dorsi/plantarflexion	Actuated	$20°/-20°$

Attachment to user's body is achieved via two elements: the pelvic module for the hip, and the cuffs for the leg segments and feet. Both are foamed and fitted with velcro straps. Most of the structure is made of aluminum due to its resistance and low weight: the exoskeleton weights only 13 kg, and its battery adds another 2 kg.

Each orthosis includes three brushless direct current (BLDC) motors (i.e., one for each of the joints), coupled to the axis of the joint. The BLDC motor used for all the joints is a Maxon EC60-100W-24V, 60 mm diameter, nominal speed 4250 rpm, and nominal torque 227 mN·m. The coupling to the output link is done via a Harmonic Drive gearbox: model CSD20-160-2AGR, with a reduction ratio of 160:1. This setup leads to a nominal speed of 26.5 rpm, constant torque of 35 N·m, and peak torque of 180 N·m, providing a high torque and low speed, both suitable to generate the movement on each of the joints [50]. All motors are driven by Advantech AZBH12A8-24 V power drivers, connected to the exoskeleton's main controller through an analog channel used for pulse width modulation (PWM).

3.1.2. Sensors

The H1 exoskeleton is equipped with kinematic and force sensors [51]. Concerning the former, each joint is equipped with a 10 kΩ high-precision one-turn potentiometer, by Vishay Spectrol, model 157S103MX, with high linearity and long rotational life. This potentiometer is used as the joint angular sensor. It is directly coupled to the output axis via a transmission belt, providing a direct measure of the joint angle.

The footplates are fitted with two force-sensing resistors (FSRs) each (Interlink Electronics 406) placed under the user's heels and toes. They allow the detection of four gait events (i.e., initial contact, flat foot, heel off, and toe off), enabling the identification of the different phases of gait.

Finally, the exoskeleton as a whole has an ON/OFF switch and each orthosis has a button that the user can press to perform a step with that leg when the step-by-step mode is activated.

The sensory data are acquired by a custom-made board (see Figure 4), one for each joint, that performs the signal conditioning, acquisition, and digitalization functions and sends the processed data to the main controller through a CAN (Controller Area Network) bus. This board's microcontroller is a dsPIC30F4013 by Microchip. The FSR data from the footplates is processed by the ankle boards.

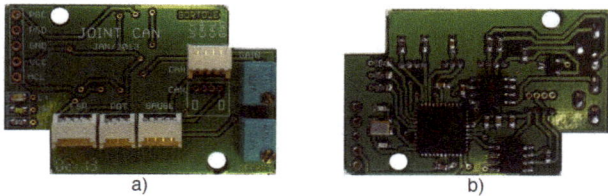

Figure 4. Custom-made boards for the acquisition and transmission of sensor data. (**a**): Top side and (**b**): Bottom side of the boards.

3.1.3. Computing Platform and Software

The main controller of the H1 exoskeleton has been programmed to run in a real-time environment on a PC/104 computer. The PC/104 main board module is connected to two Diamond Systems Corporation DMM-32X-AT acquisition boards, with 32 analog input channels (16 bits each, unused), and 4 analog output channels (8 bits each, used to drive 6 motors); a UDP communication board (Advantech PCM-363); a CAN communication board (C2-104); and an Advantech PCM-3910 power supply module.

Figure 5 shows how the sensors, actuators (motors), and electronics (both custom-made and stock boards) fit together to enable the movement of each leg. The PC/104 computer is shared by both orthoses. The UDP module is used to connect the exoskeleton to the REMOVI PBWS subsystem and a PC that the practitioner can use to control and monitor the therapy session.

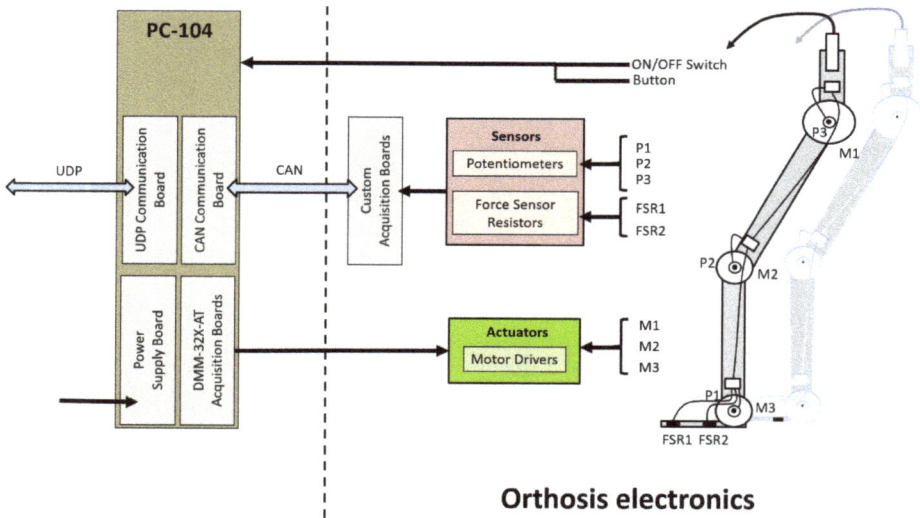

Figure 5. H1 exoskeleton electronics architecture. UDP: User Datagram Protocol.

All the exoskeleton software was implemented using Simulink. The trajectories designed for the H1 match a normalized gait pattern, provided by the *Departamento de Salud y Rendimiento Humano* of INEF by measuring 29 healthy female and 33 healthy male individuals walking slowly (around 0.25 m/s) using a VICON photogrammetry system. The resulting gait is depicted in Figure 6, with trajectories for ankle, knee, and hip.

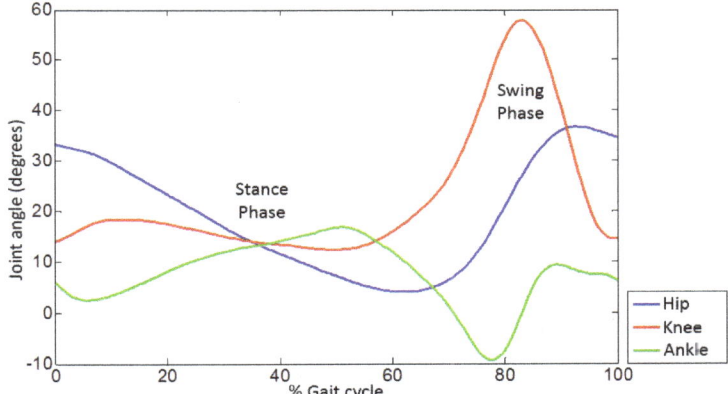

Figure 6. Ankle, knee and hip trajectories for the gait pattern.

These trajectories assume symmetry between both legs and are stored in tables used by a pattern generator module to produce a gait cycle. To implement a continuous gait they play cyclically and simultaneously for both legs, with a 50% offset between them—the normal behavior for a healthy gait [45]. This offset is shown in Figure 7, which depicts only the knee joint for the sake of clarity.

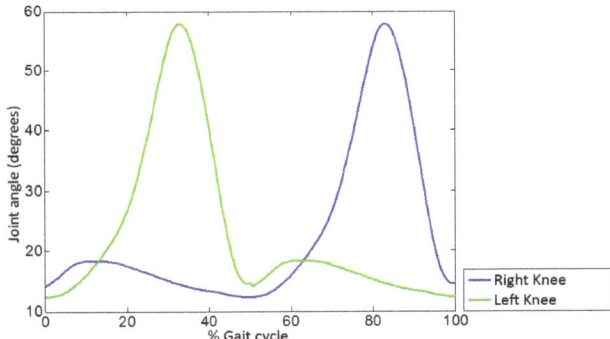

Figure 7. Gait pattern offset.

The pattern generator module supports two modes: step-by-step and continuous gait. In both of them the exoskeleton can change its speed from 0.12 to 0.28 m/s.

In the step-by-step mode, the user can perform each step independently by pressing the corresponding button. Each press induces a gentle oscillation movement in the advancing leg that translates into a single step, while the other limb moves slightly to ensure stability. Both movements stop when the advancing leg finally reaches the ground plane. This way, the patient can control pace themselves.

In the continuous gait mode, the gait pace is set and maintained. The movement is not stopped, with both legs performing the full cycle without stops between steps.

When gait is not induced (start, stop, and end of exercise) the H1 exoskeleton assumes a forced standing position, with hip, knee, and ankle at $0°$.

We implemented a finite-state machine to change between modes with five possible states (lock, left, right, left-stop, and right-stop). The output of this machine tells the pattern generator the selected mode. This translates to the following conditions:

- Always starts at the lock state; after the user has fitted the exoskeleton and activated it, the H1 stays in the forced standing position. This avoids a fall due to an involuntary movement by the patient.
- If the continuous gait mode is selected, the session starts with the right leg (to improve the learning curve of the system). This mode uses the left and right states that, when strung together, create a continuous pattern.
- If the step-by-step mode is selected, the patient can choose which leg to start with. This mode uses the left-stop and right-stop states, which generate a split pattern.
- Modes can be changed without first reaching the lock state. The system waits until the current state is finished, and then switches to a state appropriate to the new mode (continuous gait or step-by-step).
- To move out of the left-stop and right-stop states, the patient must press one of the buttons.

To avoid sudden changes in joint positions while shifting modes (lock, continuous, and step-by-step), the maximum difference between joint angular references is set to 3°, which translates into a gentle and controlled movement.

Modes are selected by the practitioner using a GUI (graphical user interface) running on a computer connected via WiFi or Ethernet to the exoskeleton. This connection and user interface are detailed later.

The software stack for the H1 exoskeleton is split into:

- A high-level layer responsible for determining the movement type, defining the joints' trajectories, synchronizing the three joints of each leg, and coordinating the combined motion of both limbs. This layer uses the stored pattern and implements the previously mentioned state machine.
- A low-level controller that maps the trajectories defined by the high-level layer to specific joint positions, implemented with a PID (Proportional Integrative Derivative) controller.

3.2. REMOVI PBWS

3.2.1. Mechanical Structure and Electromechanical Elements

The REMOVI PBWS must support patients of similar size and weight to those allowed by the H1 exoskeleton: 1.60 m to 1.90 m height and up to 120 kg weight (including the weight of both the patient and the exoskeleton). Again, these parameters cover more than 95% of the target population [48]. In this case the height is especially important for the design, since the arms' final positions must leave a clear walking area in front of the patient. Additionally, the wheelchair-to-standing position transfer process needs to be safe and progressive in order for the users not to feel that they are under risk of falling before or during this process. The proposed mechanism has a gentle upwards trajectory that is nonetheless fast enough to avoid anxiety due to the feeling of instability while being raised.

To maximize the feeling of safety provided by REMOVI, this module uses a built-in harness that spans from thorax to perineum and bears the weight of both the user and the H1 exoskeleton. This harness is suspended using a symmetric mechanism in the transverse plane (Figure 8). This setup increases the stability and balance of the patient's upper body and favors the weight transition from one leg to the other during gait. The REMOVI module also has a wheeled base with two frontal driving wheels, actuated by two direct current (DC) 24 V motors and two rear free wheels. A central column with two turning arms is in charge of the transference from the wheelchair to the standing position and vice versa. These supporting arms are actuated by a 24 V DC linear actuator and also perform the partial body weight support function. There are two hooks at the end of these arms to which the harness and force sensors are fixed.

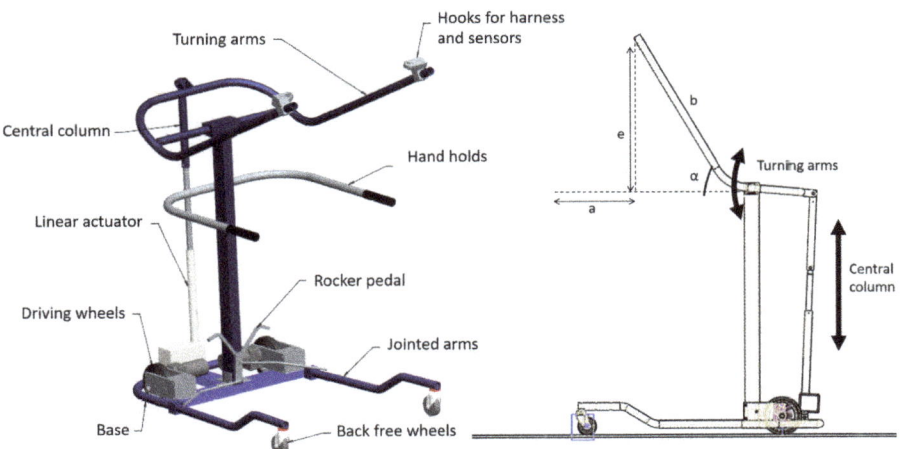

Figure 8. REMOVI mechanical structure.

The turning arms' trajectories produce two combined movements: elevation (e) and approach (a). Both are shown in Figure 8, and the relationship between them is characterized as follows (where b is the arm's length):

$$e = b \cdot \sin \alpha, \tag{1}$$

$$a = b \cdot (1 - \cos \alpha). \tag{2}$$

The wheelchair-to-standing transference can be characterized as two different phases, depicted in Figure 9. Phase I is dominated by elevation, while the opposite happens in phase II, where the approach component grows more quickly. This two-phase transference was designed to reduce the risk of falling and avoid the wheelchair being dragged.

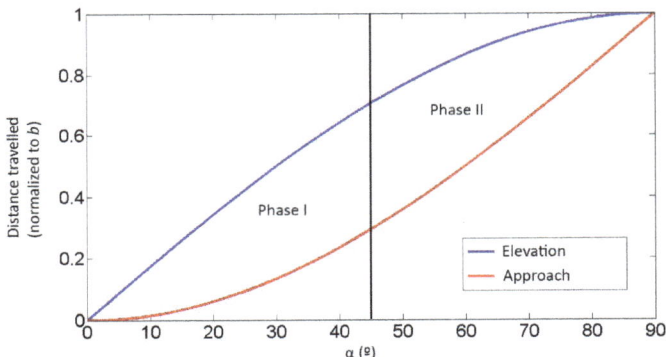

Figure 9. REMOVI mechanical structure.

For the harness, after a careful study of several solutions, we selected a thorax and groin Biodex model. Its ergonomics and, more importantly, its capacity to properly distribute weight were the deciding factors. This last feature can be used to avoid having high-pressure points that could disturb the user or even produce sores. This harness can be adjusted to different sizes and thorax perimeters, covering the desired target population.

For this transference process and the weight support modulation we chose a Linak LA345100+0L300041 24 V actuator that can push up to 5000 N, pull up to 4000 N, and has a maximum lifting speed of 10 mm/s with a stroke length of 300 mm. To measure the arms' angular positions, a potentiometer is affixed to the axis that joins them.

To be capable of self-propulsion, the REMOVI is equipped with two DC Kelvin K80-63.105 24 V tractor motors with a reduction ratio of 53.3:1 and a torque factor of 38.9. The nominal torque is 6.61 N·m, the speed is 69 rpm, and the power 50 W. Put together, they are strong enough to move both platform and user. Each motor's axis is coupled to an HEDS-5540A11 encoder with a resolution of 500 pulses per lap, tasked with measuring the PBWS speed so it can be controlled.

3.2.2. Sensors

The hooks on the ends of the REMOVI arms also contain two AMTI FS6-500 triaxial force sensors. These sensors can measure force in the X, Y, and Z axes: up to 2200 N for the X axis, and up to 1100 N for the Y and Z axes. These thresholds are sufficient for an expected maximum user weight of 100 kg. The data retrieved by these sensors (X, Y, and Z) are used to monitor the interaction between the user and the REMOVI PBWS during the elevation process and evaluate the swinging produced during the displacement of the whole system once the user is supported. The arms' angular positions (α) are measured with a potentiometer affixed to the axis that connects them.

Figure 10 shows how the relevant force components are extracted, using the following equations:

$$F_{weight} = F_r \cdot \cos(\sigma + \theta_0 - \alpha), \quad (3)$$

$$F_{advance} = F_r \cdot \sin(\sigma + \theta_0 - \alpha), \quad (4)$$

$$F_{lateral} = F_x, \quad (5)$$

$$\cos(\sigma) = F_z / F_r. \quad (6)$$

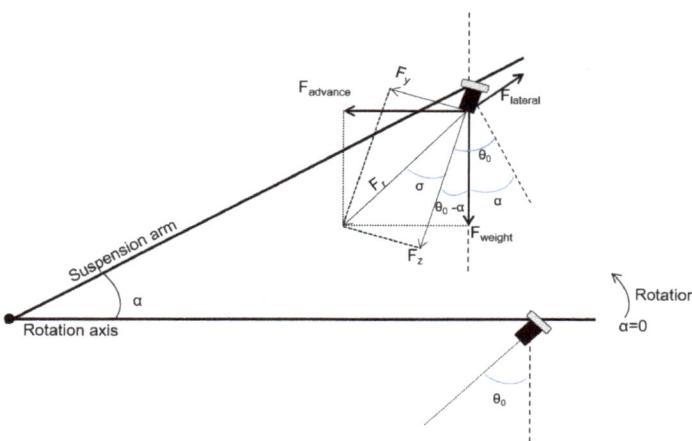

Figure 10. Force component extraction from the sensor measurements.

The three calculated components are used to determine the weight supported by the structure (to calibrate the partial suspension percentage), the forward advance, and the lateral movements (for balancing purposes). These equations are implemented in a software data acquisition block.

In addition to these forces, in order to properly characterize the interaction between the user (and the H1 they wear) and the REMOVI system, it is paramount to measure the distance between the patient and the platform itself. The advance speeds of the H1 exoskeleton and the REMOVI PBWS can be programmed so that they match each other, but in practice this is not enough to maintain an optimal relative position between both: slightly higher or lower resistance and contribution to movement by the patient, turns, stops, changes in pace and small differences in gait produce errors that add up and must be corrected. Therefore, it is necessary to monitor the real speeds of both modules dynamically, implementing a feedback loop that maintains a proper distance.

To measure this separation we have used an ultrasound UNDK 30U6103/S14 module, with a range between 100 and 700 mm and a 3 mm resolution. This sensor is placed in the uppermost part of the central column, pointing to the user's waist. The measured analog signal is sent to the on-board computer (another PC/104, different from the one on the H1 exoskeleton) that regulates the REMOVI speed so it acts as a slave subsystem to the exoskeleton (master), adapting the PBWS's speed to the user's pace. To measure the PBWS displacement speed, each DC motor's axis is coupled to an HEDS-5540A11 encoder with a resolution of 500 pulses per lap, whose data are also sent to this PC/104.

Finally, the REMOVI is also equipped with a joystick that provides manual control for the subsystem's movements, if desired.

3.2.3. Computing Platform and Software

Like the H1 controller, the REMOVI software runs in a real-time environment on a PC/104 computer and was programmed using Simulink. The PC/104 main board module is connected to a Diamond Systems Corporation DMM-32X-AT acquisition board (whose input channels are connected to all the sensors and three of its four output channels are used to control the motors through two custom drivers); a UDP communication board (Advantech PCM-363); and an Advantech PCM-3910 power supply module. The force sensors are also routed trough a Sensorex 3310 signal conditioner, since they need a stable energy supply and their signals must be amplified and filtered before the PC/104 can process them. This architecture is depicted in Figure 11. Again, the UDP module is used to connect the exoskeleton to the REMOVI PBWS module and the therapist's computer.

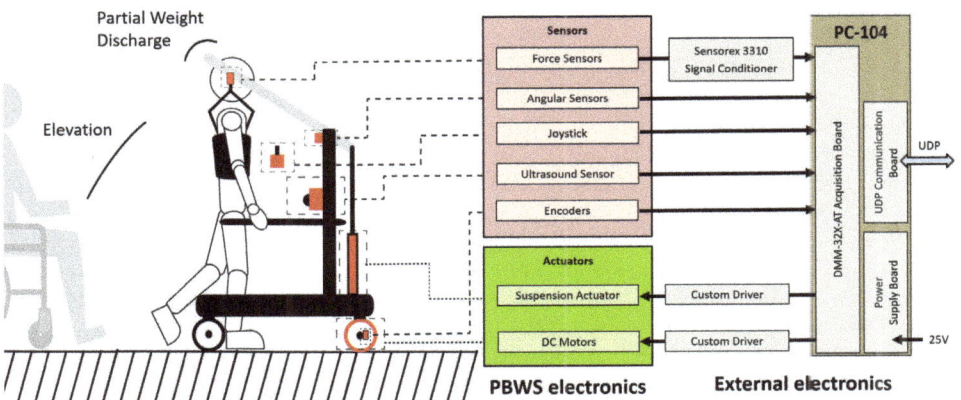

Figure 11. REMOVI electronics architecture. PBWS: partial body weight support.

The synchronization between the H1 exoskeleton and the REMOVI PWBS is achieved through a feedback loop (implemented using Matlab's Fuzzy Logic Toolbox) that controls the REMOVI speed. The input to this loop is the distance retrieved by the ultrasound sensor. The accepted range goes from 0 to 100 cm. We have defined three possible zones (near, optimal, and far distance) including this range and three corresponding input membership functions (Figure 12):

- Near zone: Z-shaped membership function with $a = 13.1$ and $b = 29$.
- Optimal zone: Symmetric Gaussian membership function with $\sigma = 40$ and $\mu = 10$.

- Far zone: S-shaped membership function with $a = 50$ and $b = 60$.

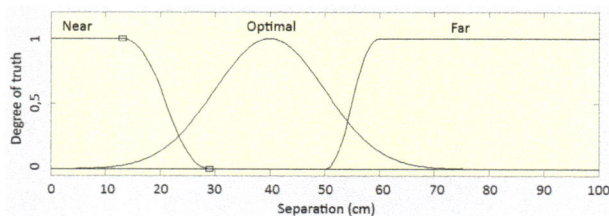

Figure 12. REMOVI distance control input membership functions.

In a similar way, we have defined three output membership functions (Figure 13) that determine three output modes:

- Stop: Z-shaped membership function with $a = 0.2$ and $b = 0.4$. Mapped to the near zone.
- Maintain speed: Symmetric Gaussian membership function with $\sigma = 0.25$ and $\mu = 1$. Mapped to the optimal zone.
- Accelerate: S-shaped membership function with $a = 1.2$ and $b = 2$. Mapped to the far zone.

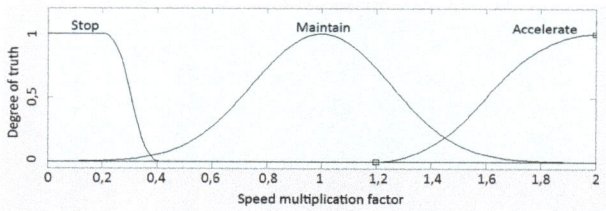

Figure 13. REMOVI distance control output membership functions.

The outputs of these functions range between 0 and 2. This factor multiplies the H1 exoskeleton speed value and applies it to the REMOVI, with the result of increasing or reducing the distance between both subsystems. The maximum factor of 2 was chosen because REMOVI's maximum speed is twice the exoskeleton's.

The elevation process is controlled by the therapist using a graphical interface (Figure 14) with three buttons: up, down, and stop. The provided interface also allows the practitioner to input the desired weight support percentage and movement speed (the same for both the H1 and REMOVI subsystems).

The suspension level can be controlled by the patient and/or the practitioner, both before transferring to standing position and during the session.

The provided software automatically manages the wheelchair-to-standing transition (through arm rotation), level of weight support, and HYBRID speed. This is possible thanks to the data retrieved by the sensors of both the H1 and REMOVI, which allow the system to adapt to the patient's weight. The forces exerted by the user are also stored for later analysis by the therapist. This way, this information is used not only for weight support control, but also to characterize the patient's gait.

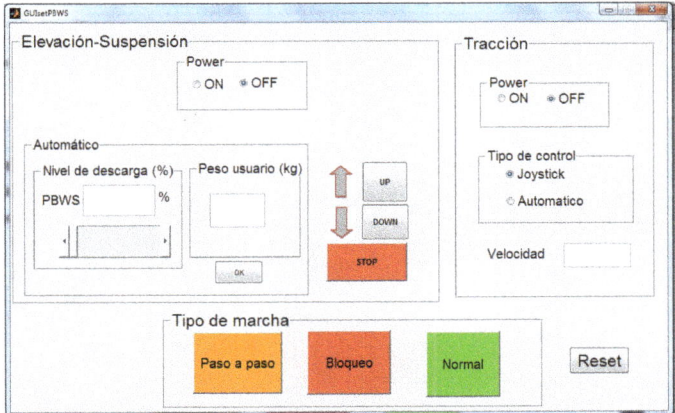

Figure 14. Therapist configuration graphical user interface (GUI).

3.3. Subsystems Communication

The H1 exoskeleton, the REMOVI PBWS and a standard computer operated by a therapist comprise a communication network that uses UDP (User Datagram Protocol) as a transport protocol. Using this network, the practitioner's computer can configure the exoskeleton and PBWS parameters using a graphical user interface (already shown in Figure 14). Both the exoskeleton and the PBWS can be connected using either cabled Ethernet or through WiFi using a router physically mounted on the REMOVI structure.

Tables 2 and 3 show the information sent by the practitioner's computer to configure the H1 exoskeleton. Tables 4 and 5 show the information sent by the same computer to setup the REMOVI PBWS.

Table 2. H1 configuration frame.

Lock	Gait Mode	Speed

Table 3. H1 configuration frame parameters.

Parameter	Value	Description
Lock	0	Forced standing position disabled
	1	Forced standing position enabled
Gait Mode	0	Continuous mode
	1	Step-by-step mode
Speed	0–25	H1 speed (rpm)

Table 4. REMOVI configuration frame.

Transfer Mode	Arms Command	User's Weight	Support	Displacement Mode

Table 5. REMOVI configuration frame parameters.

Parameter	Value	Description
Transfer Mode	0	Therapist manually controls elevation
	1	Therapist uses automatic elevation
Arms Command	0	Move arms upwards
	1	Move arms downwards
	2	Stop arms movement
User's Weight	0–100	User's weight in kg
Support	0–100	Percentage of support to apply
Displacement Mode	0	Therapist uses the joystick to manually move the system
	1	Therapist uses automatic displacement

The H1 exoskeleton also sends its speed data to the REMOVI PBWS, since the latter needs to adapt its speed to the former's. These data are sent using the frame described in Tables 6 and 7.

Table 6. H1 to REMOVI data frame.

Advance	Speed

Table 7. H1 to REMOVI data frame parameters.

Parameter	Value	Description
Advance	0	H1 and REMOVI disabled
	1	H1 and REMOVI enabled
Speed	0–3	H1 speed (m/s)

The H1 exoskeleton sends the data needed to properly monitor and control the session to the therapist's computer (Tables 8 and 9). These data are used to compare the actual position of the exoskeleton with the theoretical angles as defined in the programmed gait pattern, and evaluate the force exerted by the patient's feet.

Table 8. H1 to PC data frame. FSR: force-sensing resistors.

Right Angles	Right FSR	Right Pattern	Left Angles	Left FSR	Left Pattern

Table 9. H1 to PC data frame parameters.

Parameter	Value	Description
Right Angles	−20 to 100/−5 to 100/−20 to 20	Measured angles (degrees) for the right hip/knee/ankle
Right FSR	0 to 5	Measured force (V) by the right FSR
Right Pattern	−20 to 100/−5 to 100/−20 to 20	Theoretical angles (degrees) for the right hip/knee/ankle as determined by the gait pattern
Left Angles	−20 to 100/−5 to 100/−20 to 20	Measured angles (degrees) for the left hip/knee/ankle
Left FSR	0 to 5	Measured force (V) by the left FSR
Left Pattern	−20 to 100/−5 to 100/−20 to 20	Theoretical angles (degrees) for the left hip/knee/ankle as determined by the gait pattern

Finally, the REMOVI PBWS also sends some data to the practitioner's computer (Tables 10 and 11). These data are used to monitor and later analyze the master–slave relationship between the two HYBRID subsystems, and the rotating arms' behaviors.

Table 10. REMOVI to PC data frame.

Force X	Force Y	Force Z	Angle	Distance	Speed

Table 11. REMOVI to PC data frame parameters.

Parameter	Value	Description
Force X	0–100	Measured force (kg) for the X axis
Force Y	0–100	Measured force (kg) for the Y axis
Force Z	0–100	Measured force (kg) for the Z axis
Angle	0–90	Measured angle (degrees) for the arms' rotations
Distance	0–100	Measured distance (cm) by ultrasounds between the patient and the REMOVI
Speed	0–3	Measured speed (m/s) for the REMOVI

4. Results

HYBRID is a single solution that provides double assistance: (a) an exoskeleton and (b) a stabilization and weight support system. Both devices are independent but work in unison. Each has its own controller and implements a master/slave relationship, with the REMOVI adapting itself to the H1's pace thanks to the distance measured using the on-board ultrasound sensor of the former.

Therefore, we must ensure that there is a proper coordination between the two subsystems so that the start process of both does not feel disjointed and there is no perceptible delay between them. On top of that, the distance between the H1 and REMOVI should not vary greatly.

To check if these aims were achieved, we measured the delay between several events. We recorded the delay between the instant the patient pressed the button to activate the joint's movement and the time at which they actually started moving. We also registered how much time passed between the H1 and REMOVI begininning to move. These experiments were performed with three healthy individuals (height: 176 ± 10 cm, age: 25 ± 2 years, weight: 75 ± 21 kg). These participants were unaffiliated with the project and did not participate in any way in the research and design process of the proposed solution. All three were in the standing position with the suspension harness fitted when they activated the exoskeleton in the continuous gait mode, displacing themselves 3 m in a straight line. This experiment was repeated three times, with a support of 30%, 50%, and 70% of their own weight, respectively.

Figure 15 shows the results for the described tests. The mean delay between the button press and the moment the joints started to move was 21 ± 71 ms. The mean delay between this event and the time the REMOVI started to move was 305 ± 287 ms. Therefore, the mean delay between the button press and the instant the user started to walk was 326 ± 293 ms.

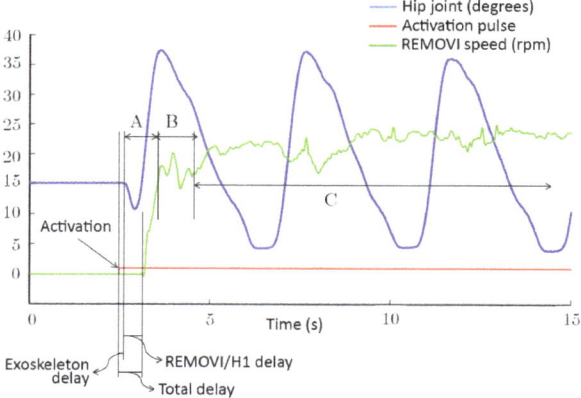

Figure 15. H1–REMOVI synchronization results.

5. Discussion

5.1. H1 and REMOVI Synchronization

After studying the data shown in Figure 15 we identified two transition periods (*A* and *B*) and a permanent regime (*C*) for the REMOVI tractor motors. *A* corresponds to the transition between the exoskeleton start and the beginning of REMOVI's movement. *B* corresponds to the synchronization process between the H1 and REMOVI speeds. During this process the developed system is using the ultrasounds to match both movements. When *C* is reached, the mean speed of the REMOVI is stable, even if there are some small fluctuations to correct positional drifts. Such drifts are usually a consequence of the user's movements, posture, and changes in pace due to lengthier strides. However, in some cases the culprits are irregularities in the floor or small wheel slippages. The dynamic range of these fluctuations was quantified as 7 ± 2.58 rpm, while the mean registered speed was 21.2 ± 3 rpm.

Taking these data into account, it can be concluded that the REMOVI properly followed the displacement induced by the H1 without losing stability, even with the added errors due to the terrain and the patient's movements. The presented values were low enough to be negligible in a rehabilitation environment, with low movement speeds. The users reported that they did not feel a sharp transition and unanimously qualified the starting process as comfortable.

Therefore, our device is also able to provide the promising "repeating without repetition" approach [52], as it permits a variation in the task of gait training. By allowing the patient to wander around the environment, we can avoid the potential loss of adherence due to the boredom that usually arises when walking on a static treadmill. HYBRID also makes the repetitive task more engaging by naturally inducing differences between gait cycles. Such variations within the task have been proven beneficial for the rehabilitation process [53].

5.2. Patient's Position

It is important to discuss an aspect of the development process that ended up being specially relevant: the position of the patient relative to the REMOVI subsystem. The design of HYBRID takes into account the anthropometric characteristics of the target users and several spatial and temporal features like the stride length, cadence, and speed, which together determine the ideal separation between the user and the PBWS. This separation must be maintained while the patient's center of gravity is kept inside the support base during both the elevation/approach procedure and the actual gait movement. Stability and maneuverability have also been taken into account. A study of the actual comfort experienced by the user resulted in the addition of hand holds to the main structure. After careful study and consideration, it was decided that the user's position relative to the REMOVI after the elevation must fit steps that advance between 20 and 40 cm at a speed of up to 0.28 m/s (covering the mean walking speed for patients with supervised walkers [54]).

6. Conclusions

This article introduces the HYBRID ambulatory trainer—a system capable of inducing a gait movement on the lower limbs while displacing at a proper pace, simultaneously providing partial body weight support and stabilizing the patient during the movement. It also features a combined elevation and approach movement that can easily, quickly, safely, and comfortably transfer the user from the wheelchair to the standing position and vice versa.

This work has taken into account the needs of motor-disabled and low-muscle-tone patients as well as the experience of clinical practitioners. The iterative development of HYBRID involved several partners and produced a two-part system that combines a lower limb 6DoF exoskeleton (H1) with a PBWS moving platform (REMOVI). On top of that, the proposed system is more than a gait trainer; it is capable of acquiring and storing the patient's data to characterize them. HYBRID is also compatible with external photogrammetry devices and other physiological parameter sensors that can synergize with the abundant captured data and characterize the user.

This system improves on the existing devices present in the literature in several ways. First of all, it combines the gait induction and weight support approaches to rehabilitation, integrating them in an ambulatory platform that can properly stimulate the proprioceptive system, posture, and dynamic balance of the patient. HYBRID also offers a novel semiautonomous elevation and transfer system. Moreover, both the H1 exoskeleton and the REMOVI PBWS maintain the features of the most popular solutions and, in some cases, improve upon them (i.e., powered ankle joints, data logging, consideration of anthropometry, gait patterns obtained using photogrammetry, a graphical user interface for the therapist). More importantly, HYBRID offers a high level of security, comfort, and ease of use—aspects paramount to the real use of a device in a clinical environment, where so often time is of the essence.

Table 12 summarizes the main contributions of this work, which is divided into two subsystems, detailed separately in this article.

Table 12. HYBRID system's main contributions.

Subsystem and Contributions	Aim
H1 Exoskeleton	
Transmission of movement to patient's joints	
Gait pattern generation	Gait induction
Bilateral coordination between lower limbs and joints	
Gait customization to patient's needs	
Forced standing position in a rigid plane	Forced standing position
REMOVI PBWS	
Semiautonomous transfer and elevation from wheelchair to standing position	Partial weight suspension
Partial weight suspension adaptable to load level	
Ease of balancing movements with upper limb support	
Increased stability in three planes: sagittal, transversal and frontal	Movement support
Increased security due to fall avoidance	

Table 13 compares the features of the HYBRID system with those of other gait trainers in the literature. In this table, the column "Interaction" specifies how the exoskeleton and the weight support systems interact with each other. The "Exoskeleton" column indicates if the exoskeleton is fixed to a platform. Finally, the "Transfer" column shows if the device has any kind of wheelchair-to-standing position transference system. From this table, it can be seen that HYBRID provides some features not present in any other published device:

- The exoskeleton is not fixed to an external platform, making a more gradual weight discharge and a greater freedom of movement possible.
- The PBWS subsystem can support up to 100% of the user's weight.
- The exoskeleton and the weight support system maintain distances using ultrasounds, without needing cables or pressure sensors.
- The system can transfer the patient from a wheelchair to a standing position and vice versa.

Table 13. Comparison between HYBRID and other gait trainers.

Device	Actuated DoF	PBWS	Support	Interaction	Exoskeleton	Transfer
WalkTrainer	6 DoF pelvis, 3 DoF per leg	Partial	Harness	Potentiometer	Fixed	No
Nature-Gaits	2 DoF pelvis, 3 DoF per leg	Partial	Harness	No	Fixed	No
SUBAR	3 DoF per leg	Only stability	Waist	No	Fixed	No
EXPOS	3 DoF per leg	Only stability	Waist	No	Fixed	No
MLLRE	3 DoF per leg	Partial	Harness	Pressure	Fixed	No
MOPASS	3 DoF per leg	Only stability	Waist	No	Fixed	No
HYBRID	3 DoF per leg	Full	Harness	Ultrasound	Not fixed	Yes

Author Contributions: Conceptualization, E.U., R.C., and J.L.P.; Hardware, E.U., G.A.-P., and R.R.; Software, E.U., G.A.-P. and R.G.-C.; Validation, E.U. and G.A.-P.; Investigation, E.U., Garcia-Carmona R.G.-C., and R.R.; Writing—Original Draft Preparation, E.U., G.A.-P., R.C., and R.G.-C.; Writing—Review & Editing, R.G.-C. and G.A.-P.; Supervision, R.C. and J.L.P.; Project Administration, R.C. and J.L.P.; Funding Acquisition, R.R. and J.L.P.

Funding: This research was funded by the Spanish "Programa Nacional de Proyectos de Investigación Fundamental no Orientados", HYBRID (Hybrid Technological Platform for Rehabilitation, Functional Compensation and Training of Gait in Spinal Cord Injury (SCI) Patients) project, reference DPI 2011-28160-C03; by Universidad San Pablo CEU and Banco Santander, under the grant "IV Convocatoria de Ayudas a grupos de investigación precompetitivos"; and by Ministerio de Ciencia, Innovación y Universidades, under the grant "Convocatoria Retos Investigación" with project reference RTI2018-097122-A-I00.

Acknowledgments: The authors want to thank the *Hospital Nacional de Parapléjicos de Toledo* (HNPT) and the *Instituto Nacional de Educación Física* (INEF) for their support in developing this solution.

Conflicts of Interest: The authors are also the developers of the proposed system and have participated in its testing.

References

1. Wirz, M.; Zemon, D.H.; Rupp, R.; Scheel, A.; Colombo, G.; Dietz, V.; Hornby, T.G. Effectiveness of automated locomotor training in patients with chronic incomplete spinal cord injury: A multicenter trial. *Arch. Phys. Med. Rehabil.* **2005**, *86*, 672–680. [CrossRef]
2. Hornby, T.G.; Zemon, D.H.; Campbell, D. Robotic-assisted, body-weight–supported treadmill training in individuals following motor incomplete spinal cord injury. *Phys. Ther.* **2005**, *85*, 52–66.
3. Husemann, B.; Müller, F.; Krewer, C.; Heller, S.; Koenig, E. Effects of locomotion training with assistance of a robot-driven gait orthosis in hemiparetic patients after stroke: A randomized controlled pilot study. *Stroke* **2007**, *38*, 349–354. [CrossRef] [PubMed]
4. Lam, T.; Wolfe, D.L.; Eng, J.; Domingo, A. Lower limb rehabilitation following spinal cord injury. *Spinal Cord Inj. Rehabil. Evid.* **2010**, *5*, 1–74.
5. Wolfe, D.L.; Hsieh, J.T.; Mehta, S. Rehabilitation practices and associated outcomes following spinal cord injury. *Spinal Cord Inj. Rehabil. Evid.* **2010**, 44–90.
6. Krakauer, J.W. Motor learning: Its relevance to stroke recovery and neurorehabilitation. *Curr. Opin. Neurol.* **2006**, *19*, 84–90. [CrossRef]
7. Reinkensmeyer, D.J.; Wolbrecht, E.T.; Chan, V.; Chou, C.; Cramer, S.C.; Bobrow, J.E. Comparison of 3D, assist-as-needed robotic arm/hand movement training provided with Pneu-WREX to conventional table top therapy following chronic stroke. *Am. J. Phys. Med. Rehabil.* **2012**, *91*, S232. [CrossRef]

8. MacKay-Lyons, M. Central pattern generation of locomotion: A review of the evidence. *Phys. Ther.* **2002**, *82*, 69–83. [CrossRef]
9. Kazerooni, H.; Amundson, K.; Angold, R.; Harding, N. Exoskeleton and Method for Controlling a Swing Leg of the Exoskeleton. U.S. Patent 8,801,641, 12 August 2014.
10. Kawamoto, H.; Sankai, Y. Power assist system HAL-3 for gait disorder person. In *Computers Helping People with Special Needs. ICCHP 2002*; Springer: Berlin/Heidelberg, Germany, 2002; pp. 196–203
11. Farris, R.J.; Quintero, H.A.; Goldfarb, M. Preliminary evaluation of a powered lower limb orthosis to aid walking in paraplegic individuals. *IEEE Trans. Neural Syst. Rehabil. Eng.* **2011**, *19*, 652–659. [CrossRef]
12. Esquenazi, A.; Talaty, M.; Packel, A.; Saulino, M. The ReWalk powered exoskeleton to restore ambulatory function to individuals with thoracic-level motor-complete spinal cord injury. *Am. J. Phys. Med. Rehabil.* **2012**, *91*, 911–921. [CrossRef]
13. Sczesny-Kaiser, M.; Trost, R.; Aach, M.; Schildhauer, T.A.; Schwenkreis, P.; Tegenthoff, M. A randomized and controlled crossover study investigating the improvement of walking and posture functions in chronic stroke patients using HAL exoskeleton—The HALESTRO study (HAL-Exoskeleton STROke study). *Front. Neurosci.* **2019**, *13*, 259. [CrossRef] [PubMed]
14. Jansen, O.; Grasmuecke, D.; Meindl, R.C.; Tegenthoff, M.; Schwenkreis, P.; Sczesny-Kaiser, M.; Wessling, M.; Schildhauer, T.A.; Fisahn, C.; Aach, M. Hybrid Assistive Limb exoskeleton HAL in the rehabilitation of chronic spinal cord injury: Proof of concept; the results in 21 patients. *World Neurosurg.* **2018**, *110*, e73–e78. [CrossRef] [PubMed]
15. Baunsgaard, C.B.; Nissen, U.V.; Brust, A.K.; Frotzler, A.; Ribeill, C.; Kalke, Y.B.; León, N.; Gómez, B.; Samuelsson, K.; Antepohl, W.; et al. Gait training after spinal cord injury: Safety, feasibility and gait function following 8 weeks of training with the exoskeletons from Ekso Bionics. *Spinal Cord* **2018**, *55*, 106. [CrossRef] [PubMed]
16. Wang, S.; Wang, L.; Meijneke, C.; Van Asseldonk, E.; Hoellinger, T.; Cheron, G.; Ivanenko, Y.; La Scaleia, V.; Sylos-Labini, F.; Molinari, M.; et al. Design and control of the MINDWALKER exoskeleton. *IEEE Trans. Neural Syst. Rehabil. Eng.* **2014**, *23*, 277–286. [CrossRef]
17. Chen, B.; Zhong, C.H.; Zhao, X.; Ma, H.; Guan, X.; Li, X.; Liang, F.Y.; Cheng, J.C.Y.; Qin, L.; Law, S.W.; et al. A wearable exoskeleton suit for motion assistance to paralysed patients. *J. Orthop. Transl.* **2017**, *11*, 7–18. [CrossRef]
18. Hyon, S.H.; Hayashi, T.; Yagi, A.; Noda, T.; Morimoto, J. Design of hybrid drive exoskeleton robot XoR2. In Proceedings of the 2013 IEEE/RSJ International Conference on Intelligent Robots and Systems, Tokyo, Japan, 3–7 November 2013; pp. 4642–4648.
19. Barbeau, H.; Blunt, R. A novel interactive locomotor approach using body weight support to retrain gait in spastic paretic subjects. *Plast. Motoneuronal Connect.* **1991**, *461*, 474.
20. Wernig, A.; Müller, S. Improvement of walking in spinal cord injured persons after treadmill training. *Plast. Motoneuronal Connect.* **1991**, 475–485.
21. Wernig, A.; Nanassy, A.; Müller, S. Maintenance of locomotor abilities following Laufband(treadmill) therapy in para- and tetraplegic persons: Follow-up studies. *Spinal Cord* **1998**, *36*, 744–749. [CrossRef]
22. Colombo, G.; Jorg, M.; Dietz, V. Driven gait orthosis to do locomotor training of paraplegic patients. In Proceedings of the 22nd Annual International Conference of the IEEE Engineering in Medicine and Biology Society (Cat. No. 00CH37143), Chicago, IL, USA, 23–28 July 2000; Volume 4, pp. 3159–3163.
23. Hesse, S. Locomotor therapy in neurorehabilitation. *NeuroRehabilitation* **2001**, *16*, 133–139.
24. Veneman, J.F.; Kruidhof, R.; Hekman, E.E.; Ekkelenkamp, R.; Van Asseldonk, E.H.; Van Der Kooij, H. Design and evaluation of the LOPES exoskeleton robot for interactive gait rehabilitation. *IEEE Trans. Neural Syst. Rehabil. Eng.* **2007**, *15*, 379–386. [CrossRef]
25. Banala, S.K.; Kim, S.H.; Agrawal, S.K.; Scholz, J.P. Robot assisted gait training with active leg exoskeleton (ALEX). In Proceedings of the 2008 2nd IEEE RAS & EMBS International Conference on Biomedical Robotics and Biomechatronics, Scottsdale, AZ, USA, 19–22 October 2008; pp. 653–658.
26. Jin, X.; Cui, X.; Agrawal, S.K. Design of a cable-driven active leg exoskeleton (c-alex) and gait training experiments with human subjects. In Proceedings of the 2015 IEEE International Conference on Robotics and Automation (ICRA), Seattle, WA, USA, 26–30 May 2015; pp. 5578–5583.

27. Stauffer, Y.; Allemand, Y.; Bouri, M.; Fournier, J.; Clavel, R.; Métrailler, P.; Brodard, R.; Reynard, F. The WalkTrainer—A new generation of walking reeducation device combining orthoses and muscle stimulation. *IEEE Trans. Neural Syst. Rehabil. Eng.* **2008**, *17*, 38–45. [CrossRef] [PubMed]
28. Luu, T.P.; Low, K.H.; Qu, X.; Lim, H.B.; Hoon, K.H. Hardware development and locomotion control strategy for an over-ground gait trainer: NaTUre-Gaits. *IEEE J. Transl. Eng. Health Med.* **2014**, *2*, 1–9.
29. Kong, K.; Tomizuka, M.; Moon, H.; Hwang, B.; Jeon, D. Mechanical design and impedance compensation of SUBAR (Sogang University's Biomedical Assist Robot). In Proceedings of the 2008 IEEE/ASME International Conference on Advanced Intelligent Mechatronics, Xian, China, 2008; pp. 377–382.
30. Kong, K.; Jeon, D. Design and control of an exoskeleton for the elderly and patients. *IEEE/ASME Trans. Mechatron.* **2006**, *11*, 428–432. [CrossRef]
31. Zhang, C.; Liu, G.; Li, C.; Zhao, J.; Yu, H.; Zhu, Y. Development of a lower limb rehabilitation exoskeleton based on real-time gait detection and gait tracking. *Adv. Mech. Eng.* **2016**, *8*. [CrossRef]
32. Guo, Z.; Yu, H.; Yin, Y.H. Developing a mobile lower limb robotic exoskeleton for gait rehabilitation. *J. Med. Devices* **2014**, *8*, 044503. [CrossRef]
33. Kuzmicheva, O.; Martinez, S.F.; Krebs, U.; Spranger, M.; Moosburner, S.; Wagner, B.; Gräser, A. Overground robot based gait rehabilitation system MOPASS-overview and first results from usability testing. In Proceedings of the 2016 IEEE International Conference on Robotics and Automation (ICRA), Stockholm, Sweden, 16–21 May 2016; pp. 3756–3763.
34. Canela, M.; del Ama, A.J.; Pons, J.L. Design of a pediatric exoskeleton for the rehabilitation of the physical disabilities caused by cerebral palsy. In *Converging Clinical and Engineering Research on Neurorehabilitation*; Springer Berlin Heidelberg, Germany, 2013; pp. 255–258.
35. Bortole, M.; Pons, J. Development of a exoskeleton for lower limb rehabilitation. In *Converging Clinical and Engineering Research on Neurorehabilitation*; Springer: Berlin/Heidelberg, Germany, 2013; pp. 85–90.
36. Bortole, M.; Venkatakrishnan, A.; Zhu, F.; Moreno, J.C.; Francisco, G.E.; Pons, J.L.; Contreras-Vidal, J.L. The H2 robotic exoskeleton for gait rehabilitation after stroke: Early findings from a clinical study. *J. Neuroeng. Rehabil.* **2015**, *12*, 54. [CrossRef]
37. De Mauro, A.; Carrasco, E.; Oyarzun, D.; Ardanza, A.; Frizera-Neto, A.; Torricelli, D.; Pons, J.L.; Agudo, A.G.; Florez, J. Advanced hybrid technology for neurorehabilitation: The HYPER project. In *Advances in Robotics and Virtual Reality*; Springer: Berlin/Heidelberg, Germany, 2012; pp. 89–108.
38. Moreno, J.; Brunetti, F.; Pons, J. An autonomous control and monitoring system for lower limb orthosis: the gait project case. In Proceedings of the 26th Annual International Conference of the IEEE Engineering in Medicine and Biology Society, San Francisco, CA, USA, 1–5 September 2004; Volume 1, pp. 2125–2128.
39. Moreno, J.; Pons, J.L.; Koutsou, A. The Rehabot-Knee Project Approach for Recovery of Neuromuscular Control of the Knee With Controllable Braces. *Int. J. Rehabil. Res.* **2009**, *32*, S112. [CrossRef]
40. Del Ama, A.J.; Moreno, J.C.; Gil-Agudo, A.; de-los Reyes, A.; Pons, J.L. Online assessment of human–robot interaction for hybrid control of walking. *Sensors* **2011**, *12*, 215–225. [CrossRef]
41. Bortole, M.; Urendes, E.J.; Pons, J.L. Integración de una plataforma híbrida para rehabilitación y compensación funcional de la marcha. In *Actas de las XXXIII Jornadas de Automática*; Universidad de Vigo: Vigo, Spain, 2012; pp. 113–119
42. Asín-Prieto, G.; Urendes, E.; Gallego, J.; Moreno, J.C.; Pons, J.L. Monitorización de la estabilidad de la marcha con exoesqueletos basada en información propioceptiva. In Proceedings of the CRIA—Congreso Regional en Instrumentación Avanzada (CRIA 2014), San Carlos, Costa Rica, 17–19 December 2014.
43. Asín-Prieto, G.; Moreno, J.C. *BioMot Project: Deliverable D4.1 – Physically Based Simulations with Partial Demonstrators I*; Technical Report; Neural Rehabilitation Group, Cajal Insitute, CSIC: Madrid, Spain, 2014.
44. Cesarani, A.; Alpini, D. MCS Organization of the Equilibrium System. In *Vertigo and Dizziness Rehabilitation*; Springer: Berlin/Heidelberg, Germany, 1999; pp. 9–47.
45. Kirtley, C. *Clinical Gait Analysis: Theory and Practice*; Elsevier Churchill Livingstone: London, UK, 2006.
46. Wiggin, M.B.; Sawicki, G.S.; Collins, S.H. An exoskeleton using controlled energy storage and release to aid ankle propulsion. In Proceedings of the 2011 IEEE International Conference on Rehabilitation Robotics, Zurich, Switzerland, 27 June–1 July 2011; pp. 1–5.
47. Meyer, P.F.; Oddsson, L.I.; De Luca, C.J. The role of plantar cutaneous sensation in unperturbed stance. *Exp. Brain Res.* **2004**, *156*, 505–512.

48. Benjumea, A.C. Datos antropométricos de la población laboral española. *Prevención, trabajo y salud: Revista del Instituto Nacional de Seguridad e Higiene en el Trabajo* **2001**, *14*, 22–30.
49. Winter, D.A. *Biomechanics and Motor Control of Human Movement*; John Wiley & Sons: Hoboken, NJ, USA, 2009
50. Riener, R.; Lunenburger, L.; Jezernik, S.; Anderschitz, M.; Colombo, G.; Dietz, V. Patient–cooperative strategies for robot–aided treadmill training: First experimental results. *IEEE Trans. Neural Syst. Rehabil. Eng.* **2005**, *13*, 380–394. [CrossRef] [PubMed]
51. Asín-Prieto, G.; Collantes, I.; Moreno, J.C.; Pons, J.L. Diseño de una órtesis motorizada de tobillo para rehabilitación de ictus con un enfoque TOP–DOWN. In *Actas de las XXXIII Jornadas de Automática*; Universidad de Vigo: Vigo, Spain, 2012; pp. 105–113.
52. Cano-de-la-Cuerda, R.; Molero-Sánchez, A.; Carratalá-Tejada, M.; Alguacil-Diego, I.; Molina-Rueda, F.; Miangolarra-Page, J.; Torricelli, D. Theories and control models and motor learning: Clinical applications in neurorehabilitation. *Neurología* **2015**, *30*, 32–41. [CrossRef] [PubMed]
53. Shea, C.H.; Kohl, R.M. Composition of practice: Influence on the retention of motor skills. *Res. Q. Exerc. Sport* **1991**, *62*, 187–195. [CrossRef] [PubMed]
54. Van Hedel, H.J. Gait speed in relation to categories of functional ambulation after spinal cord injury. *Neurorehabil. Neural Repair* **2009**, *23*, 343–350. [CrossRef] [PubMed]

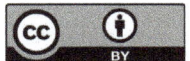 © 2019 by the authors. Licensee MDPI, Basel, Switzerland. This article is an open access article distributed under the terms and conditions of the Creative Commons Attribution (CC BY) license (http://creativecommons.org/licenses/by/4.0/).

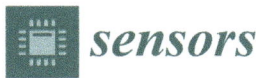

Article

Human–Robot–Environment Interaction Interface for Smart Walker Assisted Gait: AGoRA Walker

Sergio D. Sierra M.[1], Mario Garzón[2], Marcela Múnera[1] and Carlos A. Cifuentes[1,*]

[1] Department of Biomedical Engineering, Colombian School of Engineering Julio Garavito, Bogota 111166, Colombia
[2] INRIA, University Grenoble Alpes, Grenoble INP, 38000 Grenoble, France
* Correspondence: carlos.cifuentes@escuelaing.edu.co; Tel.: +57-031-668-3600

Received: 11 April 2019; Accepted: 27 June 2019; Published: 30 June 2019

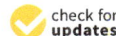

Abstract: The constant growth of the population with mobility impairments has led to the development of several gait assistance devices. Among these, smart walkers have emerged to provide physical and cognitive interactions during rehabilitation and assistance therapies, by means of robotic and electronic technologies. In this sense, this paper presents the development and implementation of a human–robot–environment interface on a robotic platform that emulates a smart walker, the *AGoRA Walker*. The interface includes modules such as a navigation system, a human detection system, a safety rules system, a user interaction system, a social interaction system and a set of autonomous and shared control strategies. The interface was validated through several tests on healthy volunteers with no gait impairments. The platform performance and usability was assessed, finding natural and intuitive interaction over the implemented control strategies.

Keywords: smart walker; human–robot–environment interaction; control strategies; shared control; gait assistance; gait rehabilitation

1. Introduction

Human mobility is a complex behavior that involves not only the musculoskeletal system but also dissociable neuronal systems. These systems control gait initiation, planning, and execution, while adapting them to satisfy motivational and environmental demands [1]. However, there are some health conditions and pathologies that affect key components of mobility [2] (e.g., gait balance, control, and stability [3]). Among these pathologies, Spinal Cord Injury (SCI), Cerebral Palsy (CP) and Stroke are found to be strongly related to locomotion impairments [4]. Likewise, the progressive deterioration of cognitive functions [1] (i.e., sensory deficits and coordination difficulties [5]) and the neuromuscular system in the elderly [6] (i.e., loss of muscle strength and reduced effort capacity [5]) are commonly related to the partial or total loss of locomotion capacities.

Moreover, according to the World Health Organization (WHO) the proportion of the mobility impaired population has been experiencing constant and major growth [7]. Specifically, nearly 15% of the world's population experience some form of disability [8], and by 2050 the proportion of the world's population over 60 years will nearly double from 12% to 22% [9,10]. These studies also report that a larger percentage of this growth will take place in developing countries [9]. Although these populations may be represented by different types of disability, mobility impairments have been identified as a common condition in elderly populations and people with functioning and cognitive disabilities [5,11,12]. Considering this, several rehabilitation and assistance devices have been developed to retrain, empower or provide the affected or residual locomotion capacities [13].

Devices such as canes, crutches, walkers, and wheelchairs, as well as ambulatory training devices, are commonly found in assisted gait and rehabilitation scenarios [14] and are intended to improve user's life quality. Concretely, mobility assistive devices are aimed at overcoming and compensating physical limitations by maintaining or improving individual's functioning and independence in both clinical and everyday scenarios [15]. Regarding conventional walkers, these devices exhibit simple and affordable mechanical structures, as well as partial body weight support and stability. However, natural balance, user's energetic costs, fall prevention and security issues are often compromised with conventional walkers [16]. Moreover, several issues related to sensory and cognitive assistance, often required by people with physical limitations, are not completely addressed by conventional devices [17–19]. Accordingly, to outstrip such problems, robotic technologies and electronics have been integrated, leading to the emergence of *intelligent walkers* or *Smart Walkers* (SWs).

The SWs are often equipped with actuators and sensory modalities that provide biomechanical monitoring mechanisms and individual's intention estimators for user interaction, as well as several control strategies for movement and assistance level control [16]. Likewise, path following modules are usually included, in addition to safety rules and fall prevention systems [20]. These features enable SWs to interact in dynamic and complex environments. The particular selection and implementation of such features can be referred to as Human–Robot Interaction (HRI) interfaces [21]. Notwithstanding, Human–Robot–Environment Interaction (HREI) interfaces are required, in such a way that they provide natural user interactions, as well as effective environment sensing and adaption while maintaining safety requirements.

In this context, the design and implementation of a multimodal HREI interface for an SW is presented. Such implementation was made to improve previous implementations of HRI interfaces on SWs, by providing safety, natural user interactions and robust environment interactions. The HREI was focused on the development of shared control strategies (i.e., natural and intuitive user interaction while multiple systems are running), as well as on the implementation of a robust Robot–Environment Interaction (REI) interface (i.e., a safety system for collision prevention, a navigation system and a social interaction system). Moreover, the interaction interface was equipped with several strategies for therapy management and supervision by a technical or health care professional. To this end, several robotic and image processing techniques, as well as different control strategies, were implemented. Navigation and human detection systems were aimed at enabling the SW with social interaction and social acceptance capabilities. Additionally, user interaction systems and shared control strategies sought to provide a more natural, intuitive and comfortable interaction.

The remainder of this work is organized as follows. Section 2 describes the existing HRI and REI interfaces implemented on several SWs. Section 3 shows the proposed HREI interface and the platform description. Since the HREI interface is composed by a HRI interface and a REI interface, Section 4 describes the systems and modules for HRI on the *AGoRA Walker*, and Section 5 presents the systems for environment and social interaction (i.e., the REI interface). Thereafter, Section 6 details the different control strategies implemented on the HREI interface, while Section 7 exhibits the experimental test conducted to assess the interface performance. Finally, Section 8 expresses the conclusions and relevant findings of this work and mentions proposals for future research.

2. Related Work

Reviewing literature evidence, several SWs and walker based robotic platforms have introduced HRI and REI interfaces. Generally, these systems are aimed at assessing the user's state (i.e., biomechanical and spatiotemporal parameters), the user's intentions of movement and environment constraints. Likewise, these interfaces and interaction systems are commonly aimed at providing effectiveness, comfort, safety and different control strategies during rehabilitation and assistance tasks. For this purpose, some sensory modalities are frequently implemented, such as potentiometers, joysticks, force sensors, voice recognition modules and scanning sensors [20]. Some of these HRI and REI interfaces are shown in Table 1, where the SWs are characterized by their type (i.e, active for motorized walkers and passive for non motorized walkers), the sensors used, the internal modules (i.e., main reported functionalities or systems), the reported modes of operation, the implemented shared control strategies and by their social interaction capabilities (i.e., specific strategies for people avoidance or interaction).

Table 1. Related works involving smart walkers with the integration of interfaces for Human–Robot–Environment Interaction.

Walker	Type	Sensory Interface	Internal Modules	Modes of Operation	Shared Control Strategies	Social Interaction
GUIDO [22]	Active	- Force sensors - LRF - Sonars - Encoders	- Autonomous navigation - Detection of user's intentions - Sound feedback	- Supervised - Autonomous	-	-
XR4000 [23]	Active	- Force sensors - LRF - Sonars - Infrared sensors - Encoders	- Autonomous navigation - Detection of user's intentions	- Free - Supervised - Autonomous	Shared walker steering on active mode	-
ASBGo++ [21,24,25]	Active	- Force sensors - LRF - Sonar - Infrared sensors - Camera - Encoders	- Autonomous navigation - Detection of user's intentions - Gait monitoring - User position feedback	- Free - Supervised - Autonomous	-	-
JARoW [26,27]	Active	- Infrared sensors - Encoders - LRFs	- User position estimation and prediction - Obstacle avoidance	- Free - Supervised	-	-
NeoASAS [14]	Active	- Force sensors	- Detection of user's intentions	- Free	-	-
UFES [16,28]	Active	- Force sensors - LRF - IMUs - Encoders	- Path following - Obstacle avoidance - Detection of user's intentions - Gait monitoring	- Free - Supervised - Feedback	Spatially modulated admittance control, visual feedback	-
PAMM [29]	Active	- Force sensors - Sonars - Camera - Encoders	- Autonomous navigation - Health monitoring	User control, path following control	Adaptive and shared admittance controller	-
MOBOT [17,30–32]	Active	- Force sensors - LRFs - Cameras - Kinect sensors - Microphones	- Autonomous navigation - Detection of user's intentions - Speech and gesture recognition - Body pose estimation - Gait Analyzer	Walking assitance, sit-to-stand assistance, nurse type	Adaptive control based on context	-
CAIROW [33]	Active	- Force sensors - LRFs	- Environment analyzer - Force analyzer - Gait analyzer	Context aware mode	Adaptive system parameters	-
ISR-AIWALKER [34,35]	Active	- Force sensors - Kinect sensor - Encoders - Leap motion sensor - RGB-D Camera	- Detection of user's intention - Gripping recognition - Gait analyzer - Autonomous navigation	- Supervised - Navigation aided	Aided user intent by navigation system	-
COOL Aide [36]	Passive	- Force sensors - LRF - Encoders	- Autonomous navigation - Detection of user's intentions	- Supervised	Shared control based on obstacles and user's intentions	-
Wachaja et al. [37]	Passive	- LRF - Tilting LRF	- 3D Mapping and localization - Obstacle avoidance - Vibrotactile feedback	- Single feedback - Multiple feedback	-	-
MARC [38,39]	Passive	- Sonars - Infrared sensors - Encoders	- Path following - Obstacle avoidance	Warning mode, safety braking mode and braking and steering mode	Shared walker steering	-
c-Walker [40]	Passive	- Kinect like sensor - RFID reader - IMU - Camera - Encoders	- Autonomous navigation - People detection and tracking - Guidance	Acoustic feedback, mechanic feedback and haptic feedback	Shared walker steering	Social Force Model for path planning

One of the most notable smart walkers is CO-Operative Locomotion Aide (COOL Aide), which is a three-wheeled passive SW [36] intended to assist the elderly with routine walking tasks. It includes mapping and obstacle detection systems, as well as navigation and guidance algorithms. Additionally, it is equipped with force sensors on its handlebars and a Laser Range Finder (LRF) to estimate the user's desired direction to turn. Although it is a passive walker, shared control strategies are achieved by granting walker control to the platform or the user.

Other passive walkers, such as those presented in [37,38], include navigation and guidance algorithms in conjunction with shared control systems. These strategies are based on sharing the steering control between the user and the walker.

Different approaches on active SWs have been developed in the past few years regarding HRI and REI interfaces [21–26,28–31,33]. These interfaces are also equipped with navigation and user interaction systems to provide shared control capabilities. Such strategies are based on granting walker steering to the user or the SW, depending on the obstacle detection and navigation systems, as well as on changing the walker responses to user's commands (i.e., some strategies are based on inducing the user's actions through haptic communication channels). To this end, user interaction systems are required to manage how user's intentions of movement are interpreted. The estimation of such intentions is commonly achieved by admittance control systems, gait analysis systems, and rule-based algorithms.

In addition, other robotic walkers have been reported in the literature, including different HRI interfaces [41–44]. For instance, the approach developed by Ye et al. [42] includes a width changeable walker that adapts to the user's intentions and environment constraints. Likewise, some REI interfaces have been presented in [45–47]. These approaches intend to assess the environment information to adapt their control strategies. Finally, regarding social interaction approaches, the *c-Walker* [40] includes a social force model that represents pedestrians and desired trajectory paths as repulsive or attractive objects, respectively. Although the *c-Walker* presents both shared control strategies and social interaction, it is a passive walker and its shared strategy is based on brakes control and shared steering of the platform.

According to the above, this work presents the implementation of an HREI interface in order to join the multiple advantages of the current HRI and REI interfaces on the AGoRA Smart Walker. The AGoRA Walker is equipped with a sensory and actuation interface that enables the implementation of several functionalities for HRI and REI, as well as a set of control strategies for shared control and social interaction. Moreover, the developed interface is equipped with a robust navigation system, a user interaction system (i.e., a gait analyzer module and an user's intention detector), a low-level safety system, a people detection system for social interaction, and a safe strategy for shared control of the walker.

3. Human–Robot–Environment Interaction (HREI) Interface

3.1. Robotic Platform Description

According to the different motivations and related approaches presented in Sections 1 and 2, this work covers the design, development, and implementation of a set of control strategies and interaction systems that establish an HREI interface on a robotic walker. Hence, a robotic platform was adapted to emulate the structural frame of a conventional assistance walker, by attaching two forearm support handlebars on the platform's main deck. Specifically, the Pioneer LX research platform (Omron Adept Technologies, Pleasanton, CA, USA), named as *AGoRA Smart Walker*, was used to implement and test the interface systems. The platform is equipped with an onboard computer running a Linux operating system distribution providing support for the Robotic Operating System (ROS) framework.

As shown in Figure 1a, several sensory modalities, actuators, and processing units were implemented and integrated on the *AGoRA Smart Walker*. The *AGoRA Smart Walker* is equipped with: (1) Two motorized wheels and two caster wheels for walker's propulsion and stability; (2) two encoders and one Inertial Measurement Unit (IMU) to measure walker's ego-motion; (3) a 2D Light Detection and Ranging Sensor (LiDAR) (S300 Expert, SICK, Waldkirch, Germany) for environment and obstacle sensing; (4) two ultrasonic boards (one in the back and one in the front) for user's presence detection and low-rise obstacles detection; (5) two tri-axial load cells (MTA400, FUTEK, Irvine, CA, USA) used to estimate the user's navigation commands; (6) one HD camera (LifeCam Studio, Microsoft, Redmond,

WA, USA) to sense people presence in the environment; and (7) a 2D Laser Range-Finder (LRF) (Hokuyo URG-04LX-UG01, Osaka, Japan) for user's gait parameters estimation.

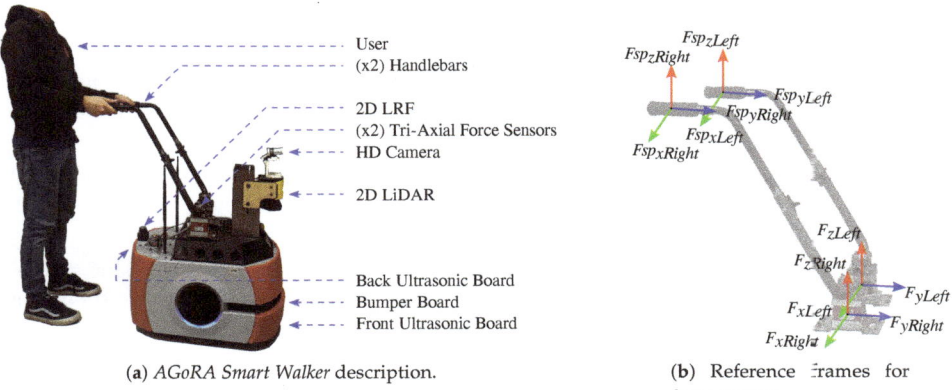

(a) *AGoRA Smart Walker* description.

(b) Reference frames for force sensors.

Figure 1. (a) The *AGoRA Smart Walker* is a robotic walker mounted on a commercial robotic platform. Several sensor modalities retrofit the walker with user and environment information. (b) Coordinate reference frames on handlebars and force sensors.

Additionally, to leverage the *AGoRA Smart Walker*'s processing capabilities, an external computer is used for running several non-critical systems. The communication with the external CPU can be achieved through the walker's Ethernet and Wi-Fi modules.

As shown in Figure 1b, the position of the force sensors on the platform's deck is not vertically aligned with the actual supporting points of the user on the handlebars. Essentially, the forces in y- and z-axis read by the sensors (i.e., F_{yRight}, F_{yLeft}, F_{zRight} and F_{zLeft}) will be a combination of the forces in y- and z-axis at the supporting points (i.e., Fsp_{yRight}, Fsp_{yLeft}, Fsp_{zRight} and Fsp_{zLeft}). The forces in x-axis (i.e, F_{xRight}, F_{xLeft}, Fsp_{xRight} and Fsp_{xLeft}) are discarded, as they do not provide additional relevant information.

3.2. Interface Design Criteria

The HREI interface presented in this work takes into account several sensor modalities and control strategies to fulfill several design requirements. The design criteria are grouped in the HRI and REI interfaces that compose the final HREI interface:

- HRI Interface functions:

    - *Recognition of user–walker interaction forces.* The interaction forces between the user and the platform are required to analyze the physical interaction between them.
    - *Estimation of user's navigation commands.* To provide a shared control strategy, as well as a natural and intuitive HRI, the walker needs to be compliant to the user's intentions of movement.
    - *Detection of user's presence and support on the walker.* To ensure safe HRI, the walker movement should only be allowed when the user is properly interacting with it (i.e., partially supporting on the platform and standing behind it).
    - *Estimation of user's gait parameters.* To adapt the walker's behavior to each user gait pattern, several gait parameters are computed and analyzed.

– *Implementation of control strategies.* To provide walker natural response to user's intentions of movement, it is required to introduce control strategies based on physical HRI between the user and the walker.

- REI Interface functions:

    – *Implementation of a robust navigation system.* To provide a safe and effective REI, the implementation of navigation capabilities is required. Such functions include: map building and edition, autonomous localization and path planning.
    – *Walker motion control.* The execution of desired movements on the walker, relays on a low-level motion control provided by the robotic platform previously described.
    – *Detection of surrounding people.* The navigation system is able to sense obstacles (e.g., people, fixed obstacles and moving obstacles) in the environment as simple physical objects. Therefore, to provide social interaction capabilities between the walker and surrounding people, it is necessary to differentiate among those types of obstacles.
    – *Path adaptation due to social spacing.* To ensure social interaction, the detected surrounding people should modify or adapt the results from the path planning system.
    – *Security restrictions.* A low-level security system is required to ensure safe interaction, even under failure or malfunction of previously described systems.

- Additional functions:

    – *Remote control by therapy supervisor.* The therapy manager should be able to modify the walker parameters, as well as to set the desired control strategy.
    – *Emergency braking system.* To provide an additional safety system, the platform should be equipped with an emergency system based on an external input that completely stops the walker.
    – *Session's data recording.* The platform should be equipped with a storage system for data recording, in such a way that the information is available for further analysis.

According to the above, Figure 2a illustrates the most relevant systems provided by the HRI and REI interaction interfaces included in our approach.

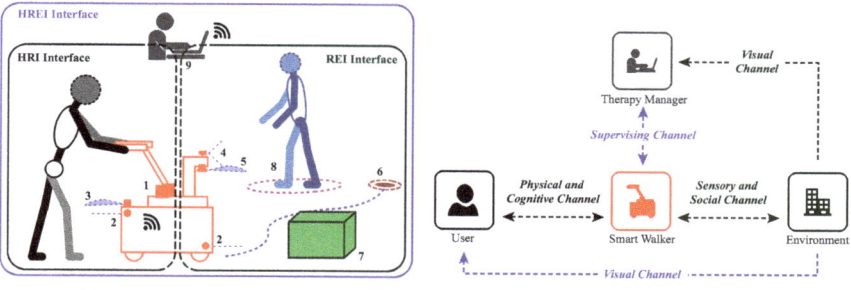

(**a**) HREI systems description.   (**b**) HREI communication channels.

Figure 2. HREI interface model and communication channels. (**a**) HRI and REI systems: (1) Estimation of user interaction forces; (2) low level security rules; (3) laser based estimation of user's gait parameter; (4) laser-camera fusion scheme for people detection; (5) laser based navigation; (6) motion control for navigation goal reaching; (7) low-rise obstacle avoidance; (8) social spacing for people type obstacles; and (9) therapy supervision. (**b**) Communication channels.

3.3. Interface Communication Channels

Relying on the different interface functions, there are some notable communication channels that provide information exchange between them, as shown in Figure 2b. The communication channels immersed over the HREI interaction are described as follows:

- *User–Walker physical and cognitive channel.* Through this communication channel, the walker's sensors assess the user's information (i.e., navigation commands, interaction forces, body weight support and gait parameters). Similarly, the user is able to sense the walker's behavior through mechanical impedance, safety restrictions, guidance, and response to navigation commands.
- *Walker–Environment sensory and social channel.* The walker's behavior is also a result of the information retrieved from the environment (e.g., obstacles and the presence people). Such information is used by the walker's systems to accomplish obstacle avoidance, safety provision, and social interaction.
- *Manager–Walker supervising channel.* A therapy manager is able to remotely assess the session data, as well as override or control walker behavior, if required.
- *Manager–Environment supervising channel.* The environment is also sensed by the natural communication channel with the therapy manager (i.e., visual supervision). Such natural sensing allows the manager to set and control the walker's behavior.
- *User–Walker–Environment visual channel.* Relying on the visual faculty of the user, the environment and walker behavior is cognitively sensed by the user. This natural communication channel takes place during the HREI loop, however it is not addressed or included in the HREI control strategies.

The following sections describe the systems that compose each interaction interface (i.e., HRI interface and REI interface), as well as the proposed control strategies.

4. HRI Interface

Based on the physical interaction between the user's upper limbs and the walker's handlebars, the HRI interface is composed of two systems: (A) a gait parameters estimator; and (B) a user's intention detector.

4.1. Gait Parameters Estimator

During gait, the movement of human trunk and center of mass describe oscillatory displacements in the sagittal plane [48]. Thus, in walker assisted gait, the interaction forces between the user and the walker handlebars are associated to the movements of the user's upper body [44].

In this sense, to implement a proper control strategy based on such interaction forces, a filtering and gait parameter extraction process is required. Consequently, the estimation of the user's intentions of movement and the user's navigation commands could be achieved with ease and less likely to be misinterpreted.

According to the above, to carry out filtering processes, a gait cadence estimator (GCE) was implemented. The GCE addresses the gait modeling problem, which is reported in the literature to be solved with several applications of the Kalman filter and adaptive filters [49]. In fact, the Weighted-Fourier Linear Combiner (WFLC) is and adaptive filter for tracking of quasi-periodic signals [49], such as gait related signals (e.g., the interaction force on walker's handlebars). Therefore, based on the on-line method proposed by Frizera-Neto et al. [50], a GCE was integrated into the HRI interface. This method uses a WFLC to estimate gait cadence from upper body interaction forces.

The two vertical forces (i.e., F_{zRight} and F_{zLeft}) are computed to obtain a final force, $F_{CAD} = (F_{zRight} + F_{zLeft})/2$. The resulting force, F_{CAD}, is firstly passed through a band-pass filter with experimentally obtained cutoff frequencies of 1 Hz and 2 Hz. This filter allows the elimination of signal's offset and high frequency noise (i.e., mainly due to vibrations between the walker structure and the ground). The filtered force F'_{CAD} is fed to the WFLC, in order to estimate the frequency of the first harmonic of F'_{CAD}. Such frequency represents the gait cadence, which is the final output of the GCE. This process is illustrated in Figure 3.

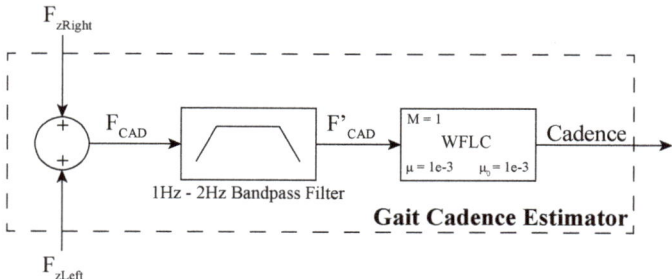

Figure 3. The Gait Cadence Estimator system takes the vertical interaction forces through a filtering process, based on a band-pass filter that eliminates high frequency noise due to walker's vibrations. Finally, the Weighted-Fourier Linear Combiner filter adaptively estimates the user's gait cadence.

According to several experimental trials, the users performed significant forces, related to their intentions of movement, along y-axis (i.e., F_{yLeft} and F_{yRight}, see Figure 1b). It was also observed that the user's navigation commands were mainly included within the y-axis forces. Therefore, the x-axis (i.e., F_{xLeft} and F_{xRight}, see Figure 1b) forces were discarded. As previously stated, the interaction force signals require a filtering process to remove high frequency noise and signal offset [50]. Thus, a fourth order *Butterworth* low-pass filter was used.

To eliminate gait components from the interaction force signals along y-axis, a Fourier Lineal Combiner (FLC) filter in conjunction with the GCE was implemented. Such integration is illustrated in the filtering system (FS) diagram shown in Figure 4. The FS is independently applied to both left and right forces obtaining filtered forces F'_{yLeft} and F'_{yRight}. Thus, Figure 4 denotes $F_{y\Phi}$ as whether F_{yLeft} or F_{yRight} and $F'_{y\Phi}$ as whether F'_{yLeft} or F'_{yRight}. The final output $F'_{y\Phi}$ of the FS is calculated as the difference between the resulting signal from the low-pass filter (i.e., $F_{y\Phi LP}$) and the output of the FLC (i.e., $F_{y\Phi CAD}$, the cadence signal obtained from each $F_{y\Phi}$ signal).

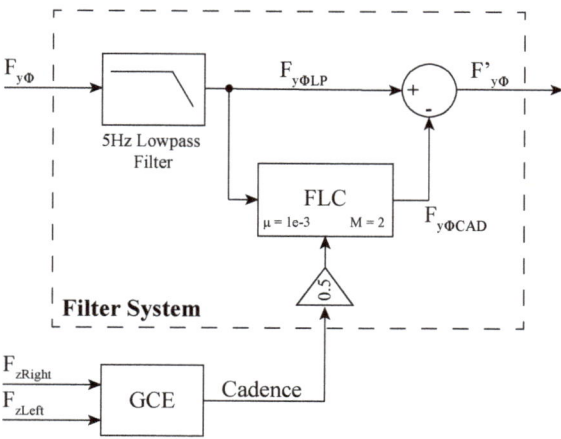

Figure 4. Filter system for y-axis forces (Φ means *left* or *right*). There is an independent FS for each y-axis force (i.e., F_{yLeft} and F_{yRight}), composed by a low-pass filter and a FLC filter.

As shown in Figure 4, the order M of the FLC filter was experimentally set to 2, and a 0.5 gain was added between the GCE's output and the FLC's frequency input. This gain was set to filter any additional harmonics produced by asymmetrical supporting forces [51]. Moreover, an adaptive gain μ of 0.008 was used.

The final linear force F and torque τ, applied by the user to the walker, were computed using F'_{yLeft} and F'_{yRight} (i.e., the y-axis forces resulting from the filtering processes) as follows: F is computed as the sum of F'_{yLeft} and F'_{yRight}, and τ as the difference between them. For instance, the F_{yLeft} signal obtained from the left force sensor and the implementation of the different filters is presented in Figure 5. The signal obtained corresponds to the readings of the force sensor during a walk along an L-shaped path. Different zones are illustrated in the figure: (1) the green zones show the start and end of the path; (2) the five gray areas denote straight parts of the path; and (3) the blue zone corresponds to the curve to the right, where a reduction of the signal is observed.

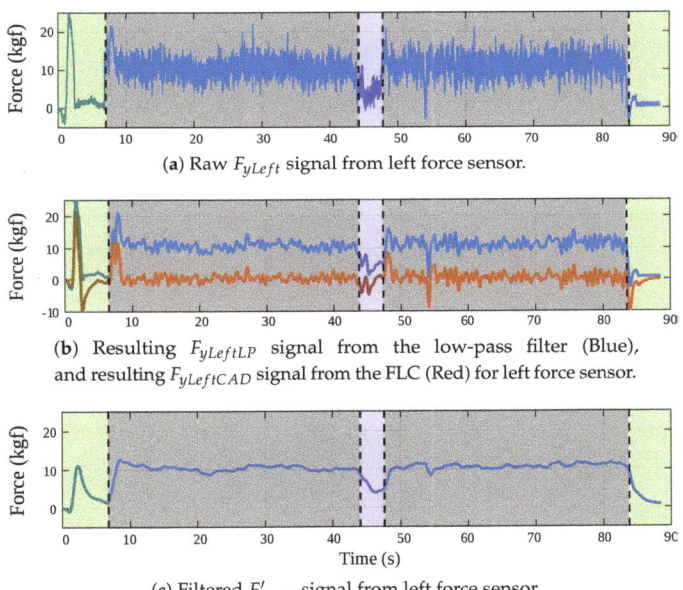

Figure 5. (a) Raw F_{yLeft} signal from left force sensor. (b) $F_{yLeftLP}$ (Blue), meaning the resulting signal from the low-pass filter, and $F_{yLeftCAD}$ (Red), meaning the resulting signal from the FLC (c) $F_{yLeftLP}$ and $F_{yLeftCAD}$ were subtracted obtaining the filtered signal without gait components, F'_{yLeft}.

4.2. User's Intentions Detector

Starting from the linear force signal and the torque signal, two admittance controllers were implemented to generate walker's linear velocity and angular velocity responses from user's intentions of movement. This type of controllers has been reported to provide natural and comfortable interaction in walker assisted gait [28], as they take the interaction forces to generate compliant walker behaviors. Specifically, the implemented admittance controllers emulate dynamic systems providing the user with a sensation of physical interaction during gait assistance. These systems are modeled with two *mass–damper–spring* second-order systems, whose inputs are the resulting force F and torque τ (i.e., the force and torque applied to the walker by the user), from the filtered y-axis forces. The outputs of these controllers are the linear (v) and angular (ω) velocities, meaning the user's navigation commands.

On the one hand, the transfer function of the linear system is described by Equation (1) ($L(s)$ stands for Linear System), where m is the virtual mass of the walker, b_l is the damping ratio and k_l is the elastic constant. On the other hand, Equation (2) ($A(s)$ stands for Angular System) shows the transfer function for the angular system, where J is the virtual moment of inertia of the walker, b_a is the damping ratio, and k_a is the elastic constant for the angular system. According to this, the static and dynamic behavior, meaning the mechanical impedance of the walker, could be changed by the modification of the controllers parameters.

$$L(s) = \frac{v(s)}{F(s)} = \frac{\frac{1}{m}}{s^2 + \frac{b_l}{m}s + \frac{k_l}{m}} \quad (1)$$

$$A(s) = \frac{\omega(s)}{\tau(s)} = \frac{\frac{1}{J}}{s^2 + \frac{b_a}{J}s + \frac{k_a}{m}} \quad (2)$$

Empirically, the authors realized that the values of $m = 15$ Kg, $b_l = 5$ N·s/m, $J = 5$ Kg·m² and $b_a = 4$ N·m·s were appropriate for the purposes of the experimental study. Moreover, k_l and k_a were used for the walker's behavior modulation. Figure 6 shows how the two FSs of the GCE and the user's intention detector are connected.

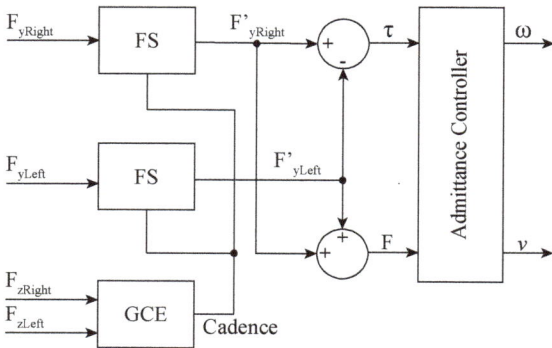

Figure 6. HRI interface system diagram.

The next section describes the implemented systems for REI on the walker.

5. REI Interface

The REI interface is composed of three main systems: (A) a navigation system; (B) a human detection system; and (C) a low-level safety system.

5.1. Navigation System

Navigation during walker-assisted gait is mainly focused on safety provision while guiding the user through different environments. According to the health condition that is being rehabilitated or assisted, the implementation of goal reaching and path following tasks is required. Moreover, such navigation tasks on smart walkers require the consideration of user interaction strategies, obstacle detection and avoidance techniques, as well as social interaction strategies. Particularly, the navigation system presented in this work considers map building, autonomous localization, obstacle avoidance and path following strategies and is based on previous developments of the authors [52].

5.1.1. Map Building and Robot Localization

Relying on the ROS navigation stack, a 2D map building algorithm, that uses a Simultaneous Localization and Mapping (SLAM) technique to learn a map from the unknown environment was integrated. Specifically, the ROS *GMapping* package for map learning was used [53]. This package is aimed at creating a static map of the complete interaction environment. The static map is made off-line and is focused on defining the main constrains and characteristics of the environment. Figure 7a shows the raw static map obtained at the authors' research center. This map is also used for the walker on-line localization. For this purpose, the Adaptive Monte Carlo Localization Approach (AMCL) [54] was configured and integrated.

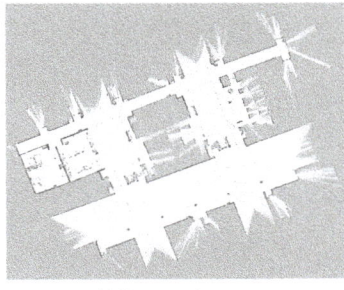 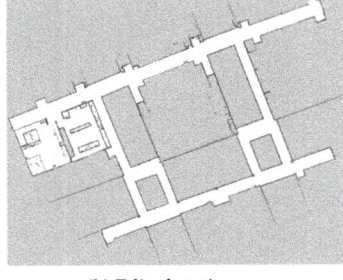

(a) Raw static map.   (b) Edited static map.

Figure 7. (a) Navigation raw static map. (b) Navigation edited static map. White means non-obstacle zones, gray means unknown zones and black means obstacles.

In general, zones such as stairs, elevator entrances, and corridor railings, among others, are defined as non-interaction zones (i.e., mainly due to the risk of collisions). These restrictions are achieved by an off-line editing process of the resulting static map. Further modifications are also required, since LiDARs are light-based sensors and the presence of reflecting objects, such as mirrors, affects their readings. As shown in Figure 7b, the map constitutes a grayscale image, therefore modifications were made by changing colors in the map.

5.1.2. Path Planning and Obstacle Detection

To achieve path planning, 2D *cost-maps* are elaborated from the previous edited map. These *cost-maps* consist of 2D occupancy grids, where every detected obstacle is represented as a cost. These numerical costs represent how close the walker is allowed to approach to the obstacles. Specifically, local and global *cost-maps* are generated. The local *cost-map* is made using readings from the LiDAR that rely on a portion of the edited map, while the global *cost-map* uses the whole edit map. Moreover, these *cost-maps* semantically separate the obstacles in several layers [55]. The navigation system integrated in this work was configured with an *static map layer*, an *obstacle layer*, a *sonar layer* and an *inflation layer* [55]. During the path planning process, the global *cost-map* is used for the restriction of global trajectories. The local *cost-map* restricts the planning of local trajectories, which are affected for variable, moving and sudden obstacles.

The Trajectory Rollout and the Dynamic Window approaches (DWA) were used to plan local paths, based on environment data and sensory readings [56]. As presented in the research of Rösmann et al. [57], this local planner is optimized using a Time Elastic Band (TEB) approach. The information of the environment and global cost-map is used by a global path planner. This planner calculates the shortest collision-free trajectory to a goal point. To do this, the *Dijkstra's* algorithm was used. Finally, a motion controller takes into account both trajectory plans and generates linear and angular velocity commands to take the walker to each plan's positions.

Figure 8 shows the trajectories planned by the local and global planner, the positions estimations calculated by the AMCL algorithm, a current goal and the cost-map grid.

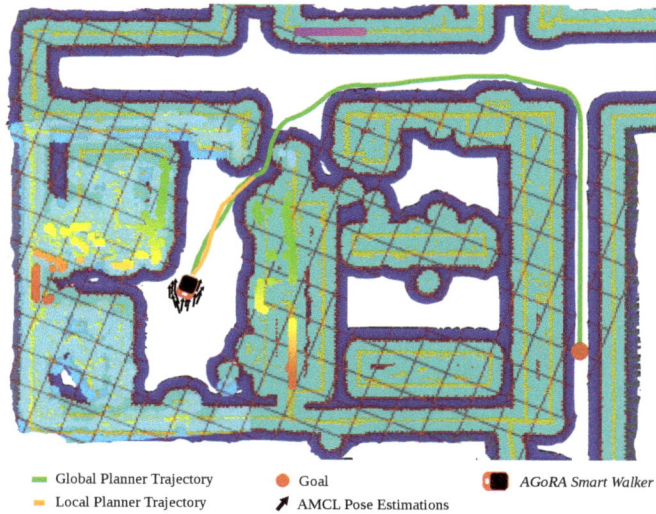

Figure 8. Illustration of a navigation task for the AGoRA Smart Walker reaching a specific goal. Green and orange lines represent local and global trajectories calculated by the path planning system. Light blue and dark blue zones represent the 2D *cost-map* occupancy grid.

5.2. People Detection System

The main goal of this module is to complement the performance of the navigation module in the distinction of obstacles regarding to people from simple obstacles (i.e., stationary or mobile objects). This distinction enables the walker with social acceptance and social interaction skills. To achieve this, the people detection system implemented in this work is based on the techniques proposed by Fotiadis et al. [58] and Garzón et al. [59]. Such approaches exploit the localization information provided by the laser of potential humans, in order to reduce the processing time of the camera data. This sensory fusion requires a proper process of calibration. Hence, an extrinsic calibration method was implemented for laser-camera information fusion. Figure 9 illustrates the methodology of the integrated people detection system.

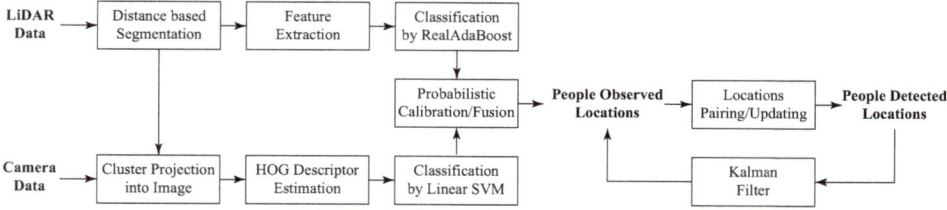

Figure 9. Outline of the people detection system.

5.2.1. Detection Approach

The people detection system begins with the segmentation of laser data into clusters, based on Euclidean distance differences. These laser clusters are inputs of a process of characteristic extraction [60]. Consequently, these features feed a classification algorithm based on *Real AdaBoost* [61], which is trained off-line with several laser clusters. In parallel, a camera based detection process starts from the projection of each laser cluster into the image frames. As previously mentioned, this projection is accomplished thanks to a calibration process that provides a set of rotation and translation matrices. Such matrices allow the transformation of laser points into the camera frame [62]. From the localization of each cluster, a region of interest (ROI) is defined for the calculation of a Histogram of Oriented Gradients (HOG) descriptor [63]. This HOG descriptor is used by a Linear Support Vector Machine (SVM), which is aimed at classifying the descriptor.

As also proposed in [58], to increase the possibilities to detect a person, the ROI is defined by several adaptive projections, resulting in a group of ROIs in which a person might be.

Both classifiers, *Real AdaBoost* and Linear SVM, are not completely probabilistic methods, since they produce probability distributions that are typically distorted. Such distortions take place as the classifiers outputs constitute signed scores representing a classification decision [64]. To overcome this, a probabilistic calibration method is proposed. The calibration of *Real AdaBoost* scores is achieved by a logistic correction and for the Linear SVM a parametric sigmoid function is used [58]. Afterwards, the outputs of each classifier are passed through an information fusion system, in order to get a unique probabilistic value from both detection methods, resulting in a decision about the presence of people in the environment.

Finally, a tracking process takes into account the previous people observations to generate a final decision about pedestrian locations. As presented by one of the authors, a Kalman filter instance is created for each detection, including those that rely out the image frame [59]. Based on each person's current and previous position, the filter uses a linear model to calculate people velocities, and consequently achieve the tracking task. A location pairing-updating process is carried out, as presented in [59]. This process is aimed at adding new people locations, updating previous locations, scoring, and removing them.

Figure 10a shows several laser clusters obtained from a LiDAR reading. Figure 10b explains the projection of the clusters into the image, where possible. Likewise, three moving people were detected out four. The laser cluster related to the non-detected person included additional points belonging to walls, therefore its detection was not achieved.

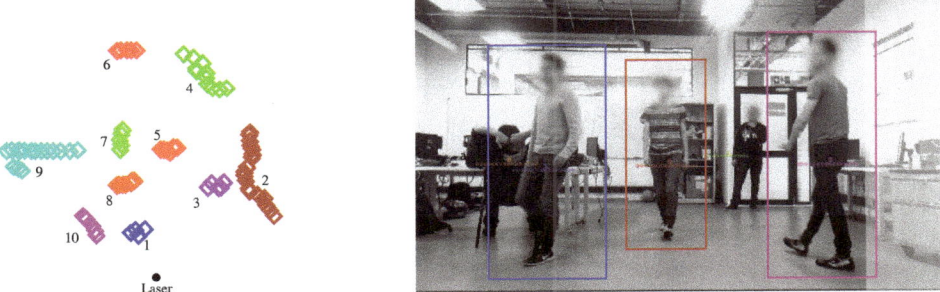

(a) Laser clusters.　　　　　　　　　　(b) Detection scenario in stationary position.

Figure 10. (a) Clusters obtained from the segmentation process of laser's data. (b) Three people detected in stationary position.

5.2.2. Social Interaction

The navigation system and people detection system are integrated to enable the *AGoRA Smart Walker* with social interaction and social acceptance skills. This is accomplished by adjusting how obstacles are understood by the navigation system. Through the modification of the navigation 2D *cost-map*, these changes are achieved. As described in the navigation system, the obstacles detected in the environment, including people, are represented as equal costs in the 2D *cost-maps*. Therefore, it is necessary to inflate the costs corresponding to a person, in order to avoid the interruption of social interaction zones in the environment. The inflation is made to match the social interaction zone of each person. This is achieved using the information provided by the people detection system, and passing people locations to navigation system. The criteria to inflate the costs are defined by strategies of adaptive spacing in walker–human interactions, as described in [65].

5.3. Safety Restrictions System

The *AGoRA Smart Walker* is aimed to be both remotely supervised by a therapy manager, meaning medical staff or technical staff, as well as to be controlled by the user's intentions of movement. Thus, some security rules were included to constraint the walker's movement.

5.3.1. User Condition

The walker movement is only allowed if the user is supporting itself on the walker handlebars, as well as standing behind it within an established distance.

5.3.2. Warning Zone Condition

The maximum allowed velocity of the walker is constrained by its distance to surrounding obstacles. A squared shape warning zone is defined in front of the walker, and its dimensions are proportionally defined by the walker's current velocity. If an obstacle yields within the warning zone, the maximum velocity is constrained.

Figure 11 illustrates the warning zone shape and its parameters that change according to the walker's velocity. The Stop Distance Parameter (STD) determines the minimum distance of the walker to an obstacle before absolute stopping. The Slow Distance Parameter (SD) determines the distance at which obstacles will begin to be taken into account before velocity limitation. Hence, if an obstacle is at distance SD, the walker's velocity will be slowed. The Width Rate (WR) parameter is the multiplying factor of the warning zone width. When an obstacle is detected within the warning zone, the velocity is limited as described in Equation (3).

$$V_{max} = Slow_{vel} \cdot \frac{D_{obs} - STD}{SD - STD} \quad (3)$$

D_{obs} is the distance to the nearest obstacle and $Slow_{vel}$ is the maximum allowed velocity when an obstacle is the warning zone. Additionally, the $Slow_{vel}$ is continuously adapted by the walker's velocity, as shown in Table 2. Such values were defined after several experimental trials, in such a way that the warning zone ensures proper stopping of the walker at each velocities range.

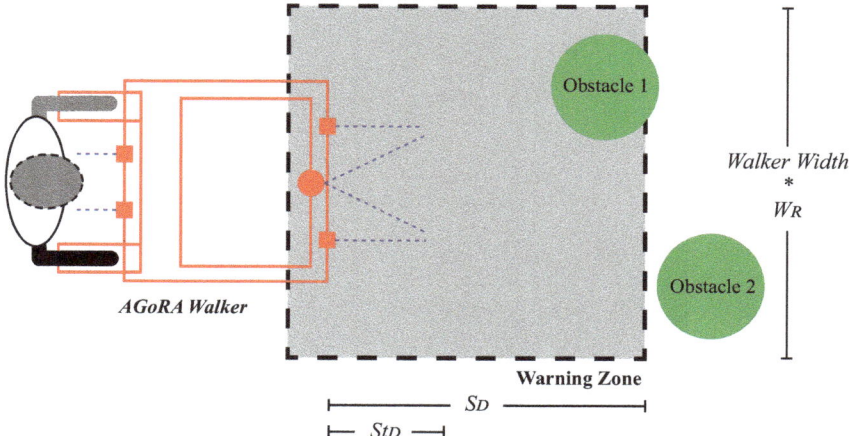

Figure 11. Warning zone shape and parameters for velocity limitation during obstacles presence.

Table 2. Warning zone parameters adaption.

Walker's Velocity (ms)	Warning Zone Parameters		
	STD (m)	SD (m)	WR
≤0.3	0.3	0.6	1.0
≤0.4	0.3	0.8	1.2
≤0.5	0.3	1.0	1.4
≤0.6	0.3	1.2	1.5
≤0.8	0.3	1.4	2.0
>0.8	0.3	2.0	3.0

6. Control Strategies

As previously explained in Section 3, the HREI interface integrates functions from the HRI and REI interfaces, in order to provide efficient, safe and natural interaction. To this end, three control strategies were proposed.

6.1. User Control

By the implementation of the HRI interface, the user is able to control the walker's motion. The gait parameter estimator and the admittance controller are capable of generating velocity commands from the interaction forces. However, the security rules keep ensuring a safe interaction with the environment. Additionally, as the therapy manager is able of controlling the walker's movement, through a wireless joystick the user's commands can be revoked or modified.

6.2. Navigation System Control

In this control mode, the REI interface has total control of the walker's movement for providing secure user guidance (i.e., the user's intentions of movement are ignored). The guidance goals can be whether programmed or on-line modified, while the navigation and social interaction system ensure safety paths. Additionally, the security rules warrant that the walker moves only if the user is supporting and standing in front of the walker.

6.3. Shared Control

This strategy combines the navigation velocity commands and the user's intentions of movement for walker's control granting. The user's intentions are calculated using F and τ, as a vector of magnitude equals to the normalized F, with proportional orientation to the exerted τ. Equation (4) illustrates the calculation of intention vector's orientation, where Max_{angle} is the maximum turn angle allowed and MET is the maximum exerted torque.

$$\theta(t)_{usr} = Max_{angle} \cdot \frac{\tau(t)}{MET} \quad (4)$$

To estimate the control granting (i.e., walker control by the user or by the navigation system), the user's intentions are compared with the navigation path, to obtain the final pose to be followed by the walker. Specifically, as shown in Figure 12, for the nearest path point (x_{nav}, y_{nav}) to the current walker position at (x_{sw}, y_{sw}), a range of possible user intentions is calculated (i.e., the range where the control is granted to the user). The positions are calculated in the map coordinate reference frame, since the navigation system generates the path plans in such reference frame.

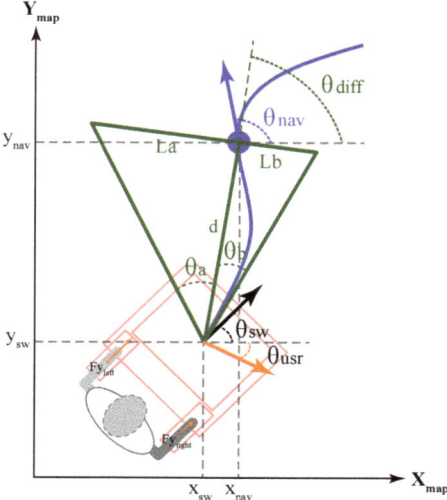

Figure 12. Estimation of possible user's intentions area.

In Figure 12, the range of possible intentions is calculated as a triangle-shaped window, which is formed by: (1) θ_{sw}, the current orientation of the walker; (2) θ_{usr}, the current user's intention of movement; (3) θ_{nav}, the orientation of the next and nearest path point; and (4) d, the Euclidean distance from the walker position to the next pose. The geometric parameters for the window formation are described in Equations (5)–(8). A window scaling factor $Wind_{width}$ is used to adapt the window area. Graphically, the window is formed by two right-angled triangles. These smaller triangles are constituted with height d, bases La and Lb, and auxiliary angles θ_a and θ_b.

$$La = \frac{Win_{width} \cdot (\theta_{nav} - \theta_{sw})}{Max_{angle}} \quad (5)$$

$$Lb = Win_{width} - La \quad (6)$$

$$\theta_a = tan^{-1}\left(\frac{La}{d}\right) \quad (7)$$

$$\theta_b = tan^{-1}\left(\frac{Lb}{d}\right) \quad (8)$$

If the user's intention of movement lies in the described window, the control is granted to the user. Otherwise, if the user's objective lies outside the area of possible movements, a new path pose is computed. This new pose is calculated to be within the area of possible movements. To this end, both x_{nav} and y_{nav} define the new pose position and the new pose orientation (θ_{nxt}) is defined as presented in Equation (9):

$$\theta_{nxt} = \begin{cases} \theta_{nav}, & if \quad \theta_{diff} - \theta_a \leq \theta_{usr} \leq \theta_{diff} + \theta_b \\ \theta_{diff} - \theta_a, & if \quad \theta_{usr} < \theta_{diff} - \theta_a \\ \theta_{diff} + \theta_b, & if \quad other \end{cases} \quad (9)$$

where θ_{diff} is estimated as shown in Equation (10) and represents the relative center of the window of possible movements.

$$\theta_{diff} = sin^{-1}\left(\frac{y_{nav} - y_{sw}}{d}\right) \quad (10)$$

7. Experimental Tests

To evaluate the described HREI interface, several performance and usability tests were proposed, regarding the control strategies previously described. The main goal of these tests was to assess the performance of every module of the *AGoRA Smart Walker*, both independently and simultaneously. Several healthy subjects were recruited to voluntarily participate in the validation study. Specifically, seven volunteers conformed the validation group (6 males, 1 female, 33.71 ± 16.63 y.o., 1.69 ± 0.056 m, 65.42 ± 7.53 kg) with no gait assistance requirements accomplished the tests that are further presented (see Table 3 for additional information).

Table 3. Summary of volunteers who participated in the study.

Subject	Age (y.o.)	Height (m)	Weight (kg)	Gender
1	23	1.76	65	Male
2	23	1.77	72	Male
3	23	1.65	62	Female
4	61	1.67	65	Male
5	23	1.72	69	Male
6	59	1.60	50	Male
7	24	1.70	75	Male

The experimental trials took place at the laboratories building of the Colombian School of Engineering. A total of 21 trials divided into 7 sessions were performed. Every session consisted in three different trials of each specific control mode (i.e., user control, navigation system control and shared control). At the beginning of each session, the order in which the modes of operation were going to be evaluated was randomized. Likewise, before each trial the volunteers were instructed in the behavior of control mode, allowing them to interact with the platform. During trials, the researchers stayed out of the session environment to avoid interfering with the tasks achievement. At the end of each trial, a data log including user and walker's information was stored for further analysis purposes.

According to the above, the obtained results under each control mode are presented in the following sub-sections.

7.1. User Control Tests

The volunteers were asked to achieve a square-shaped trajectory by following several landmarks. Figure 13a illustrates the reference trajectory to be followed by the participants and Figure 13b illustrates the achieved trajectories by the participants. Under this control mode, the only active systems were those corresponding to the HRI interface. The trajectory was aimed at assessing the capabilities of the interface to respond to the users' intentions of movement and adapt to their gait pattern. Specifically, the gait parameter estimator was responsible for acquiring and filtering the force and torque signals due to the physical interaction between the walker and the user. As an explanatory result, Figure 14a shows the filtered signals regarding to force and torque for subject 1. The user's intentions detector was in charge of generating the linear and angular speed control signals of the walker. Figure 14b shows the speed signals for subject 1. Similarly, the low level security system was running in parallel, in such a way that collisions were avoided. Specifically, no collisions took place during these trials.

During the execution user control trials, higher differences were encountered between the ideal and the achieved paths at the trajectory corners. Accordingly, the 90-degree turns were more difficult to accomplish by the participants, as the *AGoRA Walker* axis of rotation is not aligned with the user's axis of rotation. However, such kind of turns should be avoided as they risk user's stability and balance. Thus, less steep turns are more natural and safer for the users.

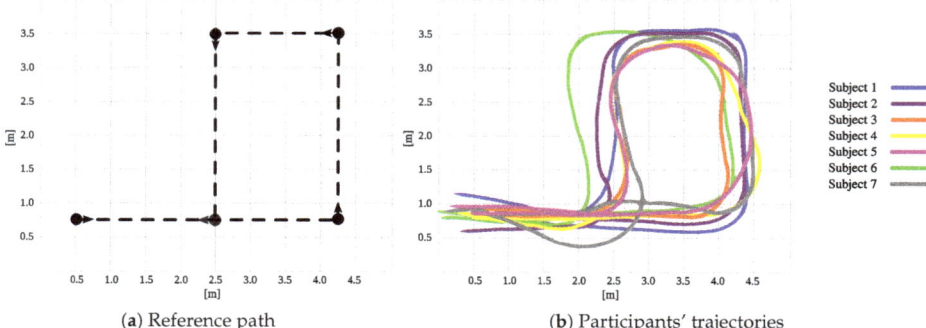

(a) Reference path (b) Participants' trajectories

Figure 13. (a) Reference path for user control tests based on a square-shaped trajectory. Landmarks and path direction were indicated through reference points at path corners. (b) Trajectories achieved by the nine participants under user control trials.

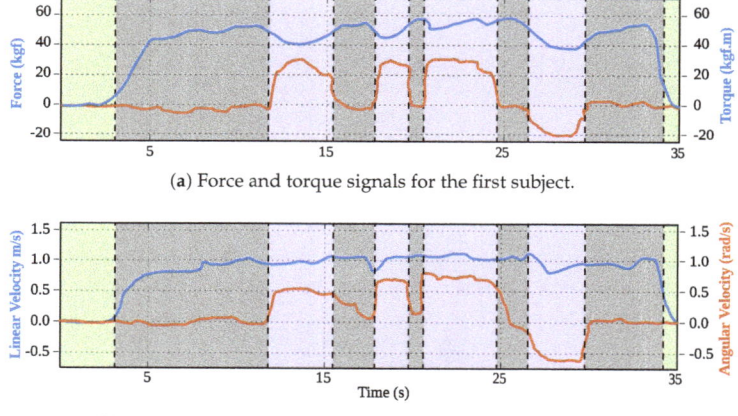

(a) Force and torque signals for the first subject.

(b) Responses from the admittance controller for the first subject.

Figure 14. (a) Force (blue) and torque (orange) signals during the trajectory for the first subject. (b) Linear (blue) and angular (orange) velocities obtained from the admittance controller during the trajectory for the first subject.

7.2. Navigation System Control Tests

To evaluate the path following and security restrictions capabilities alongside the people detection system, a preliminary guidance trial with one subject was performed in presence of people. The volunteer user was guided through a random path previously programmed, while overcoming both regular and people obstacles in the environment. Additionally, the navigation system was configured with: (1) minimum turning radius of 15 cm, to avoid steeped curves planning; (2) local planner frequency of 25 Hz; (3) global planner frequency of 5 Hz; and (4) maximum linear velocity of 0.3 m/s and maximum angular velocity of 0.2 rad/s.

Figure 15 illustrates the carried out test in three different states. The first state shows the planned trajectory according to the initial environment sense, as shown in Figure 15a. The second state in Figure 15b presents an update in the trajectory due to new people locations. Although the most proximate person to the walker is not detected by the camera, laser readings allows the person's position tracking and therefore its detection. Finally, Figure 15c illustrates the avoiding of another person, while continuing with the guidance task.

In addition to the above, the guiding capability of the navigation system was also validated on the seven volunteers who participated in the study. Specifically, the predefined path goals presented in Figure 16 were configured in the navigation system to form a desired trajectory. The reference trajectory was designed to be similar to the reference path used for the user control trials. However, the trajectory corners were designed as soft turn curves, in such a way that the user's balance and stability were not compromised. During the seven trials, no significant differences were encountered in the achieved trajectories, no collisions took place and the mean guidance task time was 53.06 ± 2.15 s. The participants were asked to perceive their interactions with the *AGoRA Walker* during the guiding task.

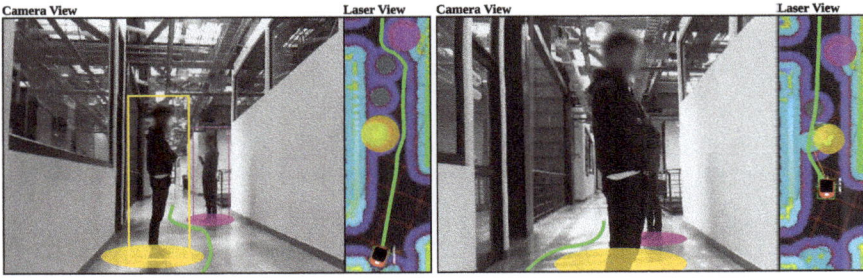

(a) Path planning overcoming two detected people.

(b) Path planning update after new people locations.

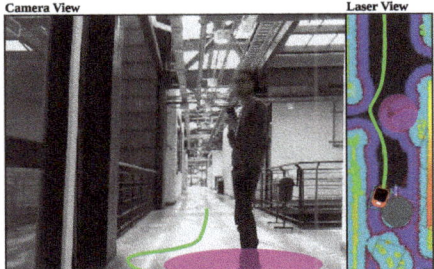

(c) Final path planning update.

Figure 15. Navigation and people detection systems during guidance task. Yellow and purple squares represent people obstacles detected by both camera and laser. Yellow and purple circles represent people obstacles only detected by the laser, as well as the obstacles costs inflations. Gray circles show old obstacles that will be removed once the walker senses such areas again. Green line illustrates the path.

7.3. Shared Control Tests

To assess the shared control performance, each volunteer was asked to follow the reference trajectory previously presented in Figure 16. Under this control mode, the participants were partially guided by the navigation system. Likewise, before each trial the volunteers were informed that their intentions of movement would be taken into account. The Table 4 summarizes main findings for each trial.

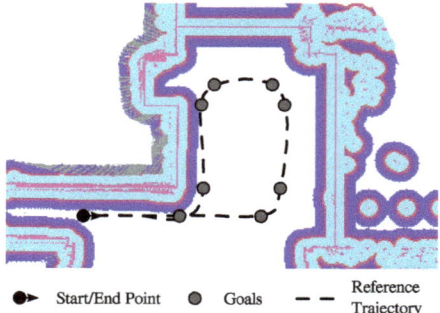

Figure 16. Reference trajectory and goals for the guiding task.

Table 4. Summary of the results obtained for shared control trials.

Subject	Achieved Goals	Task Time (s)	Mean Linear Speed (m/s)	Percentage of User Control (%)
1	10	63.94	0.34	69.19
2	10	71.46	0.34	71.63
3	10	48.38	0.46	53.66
4	10	83.45	0.23	62.55
5	10	64.54	0.34	68.25
6	8	80.8	0.21	73.99
7	10	60.29	0.37	67.71

The results presented in Table 4 suggest proper capabilities of the shared control strategy to effectively guide the participants through a specific trajectory. Six subjects achieved the full reference path by reaching its ten intermediate goals. Specifically, one subject did not complete the task by only reaching eight goals. This result is due to a random false obstacle perceived at the ninth goal, resulting in the blocking of the path planning module. Regarding the task completion times, the mean task time obtained for all the participants was 67.55 ± 11.25 s. The differences among these times is mainly supported by the fact that the linear speed was totally controlled by the user intentions of movement. Accordingly, the obtained mean linear speed was 0.33 ± 0.07 m/s. Finally, to evaluate the control granting behavior under this mode, the percentage of user control was estimated. This ratio was calculated taking into account the total time of user control and the overall task time. A mean percentage of $66.71 \pm 6.26\%$ was obtained. The user control occurred mainly in the straight segments of the trajectory, since at the trajectory curves the users' intentions of movement did not completely matched to the planned path.

7.4. Questionnaires Responses

To qualitatively assess the interactions between the participants and the *AGoRA Walker*, at the end of each trial, the volunteers were asked to fill out a usability questionnaire to obtain instant perceptions of the mode of operation. The participants were also encouraged to highlight perceptions regarding the interaction with the smart walker. Regarding the perception questionnaire, based on the UTAUT models in [66,67], an acceptance and usability questionnaire was designed. The questionnaire was adapted to be relevant to the interaction with the AGoRA Walker (see Table 5 for further details).

Table 5. Acceptance and usability questionnaire used in the study.

No.	Question
Q1	I think the robotic device makes me feel safe
Q2	I think the robotic device was easy to use
Q3	I think most people would learn to use this device quickly, it is intuitive
Q4	I think the device guides me well
Q5	I think my experience interacting with the device was natural
Q6	I think my experience interacting with the device was intuitive
Q7	I think my experience interacting with the device was stressful.
Q8	In this session, I felt that I had control of the device
Q9	In this session, I felt that the device had the control of the path to be followed
Q10	In this session, I felt that the device control was shared with me

The Likert data obtained from the acceptance and usability questionnaires were aimed at assessing the participants' perceptions of the interaction with the *AGoRA Walker*. For analysis purposes, the answers from Questions Q1–Q4 were grouped into a single category (C1), since they evaluated the attitude towards the device and the expected performance. Similarly, the answers from Questions Q5–Q7 were grouped into another category (C2), as they evaluated the perceived effort and anxiety of the interaction with the device. Finally, Questions Q8–Q10 were aimed at assessing the behavior perception of each control mode. However, the answers from these question were independently analyzed, in order to find differences between them. The questionnaire responses are presented in Figure 17, illustrating the percentage of opinions in each category (i.e., C1 and C2), as well as in Questions Q8–Q10 for each Likert item.

Relying on the questionnaire responses for Categories C1 and C2, a direct measure of the interaction perception in the experimental sessions can be obtained. Consequently, resembling survey answers were obtained under each control mode with major positive distributions. These results might suggest safe, natural and intuitive interactions perceived by the volunteers who participated in the study. Moreover, some participants stated additional comments regarding to the navigation control mode. Specifically, the volunteers suggested that at specific trajectory points the device stopped, in such a way that the path following task was not very comfortable. These impressions occurred at several trajectory goals, since the navigation system was configured to reach them at specific orientations.

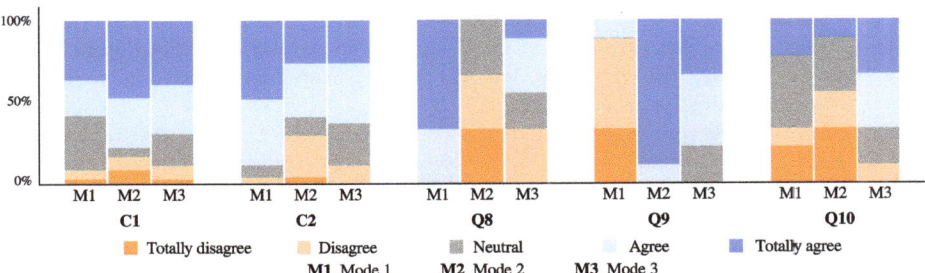

Figure 17. Acceptance and usability questionnaire results: Mode 1, user control; Mode 2. navigation system control; Mode 3, shared control.

To analyze the participants' behavior perception under each control mode, the responses from Questions Q8–Q10 were statistically analyzed. As found in [68,69], Mann–Whitney–Wilcoxon (MWW) tests have shown optimal results comparing Likert data for small sample sizes MWW. Therefore, the MWW test was used to assess differences in the perception of each control mode. Specifically, Table 6 summarizes the *p* values obtained for each paired test between control modes (i.e., Mode 1, user control; Mode 2, navigation system control; and Mode 3, shared control).

Table 6. Mann–Whitney–Wilcoxon p values for paired tests among Q8, Q9 and Q10. p values in bold illustrate significant differences encountered, meaning $p \leq 0.05$.

Question	Mode 1 vs. Mode 2	Mode 1 vs. Mode 3	Mode 2 vs. Mode 3
Q8	**0.02**	**0.02**	**0.05**
Q9	**0.02**	**0.02**	0.08
Q10	0.37	0.136	**0.04**

As can be seen in Table 6 and Figure 17, significant differences were encountered among all participants responses for Question Q8. Such outcome may suggest that all participants perceived the ability of the interface to respond to their intentions of movement. Likewise, responses for question Q9 showed significant differences between two paired tests (i.e., Mode 1 vs. Mode 2 and Mode 1 vs. Mode 3), indicating that participants perceived modifications in the walker behavior. Finally, regarding Question Q10, a significant difference was only obtained for paired test between Mode 2 and Mode 3. Such behavior might be supported by the fact that both navigation system control and user control work together under the shared control mode.

8. Conclusions and Future Work

An HREI interface, composed by HRI and REI interfaces, was developed and implemented on a robotic platform for walker assisted gait. The robotic platform was equipped with two handlebars for forearm support and several sensory modalities, in order to emulate the performance and capabilities of an SW. Within the HREI interface design criteria, the following functions are found: estimation of user's intentions of movement, providing of a safe and natural HRI interaction, implementation of a navigation system alongside a people detection system for social interaction purposes, and the integration of a set of control strategies for intuitive and natural interaction.

To validate the platform performance and interaction capabilities, several preliminary tests were conducted with seven volunteer users with no gait requirements reported. Specifically, data were collected from 21 trials divided into seven sessions, where all participant interacted with each control mode. Regarding the user control mode, a squared-shaped trajectory was proposed to be followed by each participant. The achieved trajectories for all the volunteers, as well as the admittance responses for a specific subject were presented. According to the participants' performance under this control mode, preferences for less steeped curves were found. Concretely, the participants did not strictly execute 90-degree turns at trajectory corners. Such behavior is mainly supported by the not aligned axes of rotation of the walker and the users. Moreover, ignoring path corners allowed the participants to ensure balance and stability during walking.

The validation trials were also aimed at assessing the performance of the navigation system in guidance tasks, as well as at evaluating the performance of the navigation and people detection systems working together. Specifically, an isolated preliminary test with a volunteer was carried out to evaluate the capabilities of the platform for overcoming environments with people, even when sudden changes in obstacles locations. In the preliminary test, both navigation and people detection systems were executed at a maximum frequency of 4 Hz, due the on-board computational limitations. To ensure user's balance and stability, the trajectory planning was configured to prefer curves with minimum turning radius of 15 cm. Although collisions and system clogging were not presented, the implementation of the REI on clinical or crowded scenarios should required higher computational resources. Regarding the validation trials with the seven volunteer users, a reference trajectory composed by 10 intermediate goals was proposed. All participants experienced the navigation system control completely achieving the reference path with no collisions.

Regarding the assessment of the shared control mode, a path following task was also proposed. Under this control mode, the participant's intentions of movements and the navigation system cooperatively controlled the platform. Specifically, the linear speed was totally controlled by the users. Similarly, the angular speed was controlled according to the shared control strategy estimations. To ensure participant's balance and stability, minimal turning radius of 15 cm were also configured. Among the participants trials, a mean percentage of user control of 66.71 ± 6.26 was obtained. Concretely, the control of the platform was mainly granted to the user at straight segments of the trajectory, since the participants' did not have exact information about the reference trajectory. According to the geometrical model implemented for the shared control strategy, more strict or more flexible behaviors can be configured by modifying the dimensions of the interaction window. Such modifications can potentially be implemented in rehabilitation scenarios in order to provide different levels of assistance. Specifically, early stages of physical and cognitive rehabilitation processes might benefit from more rigorous interaction windows, ensuring a higher percentage of control of the navigation system.

A qualitative assessment of the platform performance and interaction capabilities relying on an acceptance and usability questionnaire was carried out. The participants' attitude towards the device, as well as the performance and behavior perception were evaluated. According to the survey responses, the participants perceived a mostly positive interaction with the platform. Specifically, the questionnaires showed natural, safe and intuitive interactions under all the control modes. Regarding the behavior perception, significant differences were statistically found between the control modes. Slightly negative distributions were found for the navigation system control for C2 questions. These questions were aimed at evaluating effort and anxiety perceptions, which where experience by some participants. Particularly, two volunteers stated that the navigation system suddenly stopped at specific points of the trajectory. Such behavior was mainly due to the system configuration to reach goals at specific orientations.

Future works will address extensive evaluations of social interactions between the walker and people in the environment, by implementing several avoidance strategies, as well as algorithms for recognition of social groups interactions. Similarly, the assessment of the interface here proposed in clinical and rehabilitation scenarios will be achieved. Specifically, validation studies will firstly be carried out on post-stroke patients as they require a lower assistance level than SCI and CP patients. These validation studies will be aimed at analyzing specific relationships between the users' characteristics and the interaction performance. Moreover, according to the the *AGoRA Walker*'s handlebars configuration, the platform might be classified as an assistance SW. Therefore, the HREI interface will be implemented and validated on a rehabilitation SW. Additional developments will seek to implement feedback strategies for the user under each control mode, in order to pursue better performance and interaction perceptions. Future works will also address the implementation of the presented interface on an SW that cooperates with an exoskeleton for gait assistance and rehabilitation. Finally, the integration of a cloud based system could leverage processing capabilities, resulting in better performance results.

Author Contributions: Conceptualization, S.D.S.M. and C.A.C.; methodology, S.D.S.M. and C.A.C.; software, S.D.S.M. and M.G.; validation, S.D.S.M.; investigation, S.D.S.M.; resources, M.M.; data curation, S.D.S.M.; writing—original draft preparation, S.D.S.M.; writing—review and editing, M.G., M.M. and C.A.C.; supervision, M.M. and C.A.C.; project administration, M.M. and C.A.C.; and funding acquisition, M.M. and C.A.C.

Funding: This work was supported by the Colombian Administrative Department of Science, Technology and Innovation *Colciencias* (grant ID No. 801-2017) and Colombian School of Engineering Julio Garavito internal funds.

Acknowledgments: This work was supported by Colombian Department Colciencias (Grant 801-2017) and the Colombian School of Engineering Julio Garavito Funds. The authors also wish to acknowledge the support from project CAMPUS (Connected Automated Mobilty Platform for Urban Sustainability) sponsored by Programme d'Investissements d'Avenir (PIA) of the French Agence de l'Environnement et de la Maîtrise de l'Énergie (ADEME).

Conflicts of Interest: The authors declare no conflict of interest

Abbreviations

The following abbreviations are used in this manuscript:

SCI	Spinal Cord Injury
CP	Cerebral Palsy
WHO	World Health Organization
SW	Smart Walker
SWs	Smart Walkers
HRI	Human–Robot Interaction
HREI	Human–Robot–Environment Interaction
REI	Robot–Environment Interaction
COOL Aide	CO-Operative Locomotion Aide
ROS	Robotic Operating System
IMU	Inertial Measurement Unit
LiDAR	Light Detection and Ranging Sensor
HD	High Definition
LRF	Laser Range Finder
CPU	Central Processing Unit
F_{xRight}	Force along the x-axis on the right load cell
F_{xLeft}	Force along the x-axis on the left load cell
F_{yRight}	Force along the y-axis on the right load cell
F_{yLeft}	Force along the y-axis on the left load cell
F_{zRight}	Force along the z-axis on the right load cell
F_{zLeft}	Force along the z-axis on the left load cell
Fsp_{xRight}	Force along the x-axis on the right supporting point
Fsp_{xLeft}	Force along the x-axis on the left supporting point
Fsp_{yRight}	Force along the y-axis on the right supporting point
Fsp_{yLeft}	Force along the y-axis on the left supporting point
Fsp_{zRight}	Force along the z-axis on the right supporting point
Fsp_{zLeft}	Force along the z-axis on the left supporting point
GCE	Gait Cadence Estimator
WFLC	Weighted-Fourier Linear Combiner
F_{CAD}	Resulting force used to estimate user's gait cadence
F'_{CAD}	Filtered F_{CAD} force
FLC	Fourier Lineal Combiner
FS	Filtering System of forces along y-axis
$F_{y\Phi}$	Representation of whether F_{yLeft} or F_{yRight}
F'_{yLeft}	Filtered F_{yLeft}
F'_{yRight}	Filtered F_{yRight}
$F'_{y\Phi}$	Representation of whether F'_{yLeft} or F'_{yRight}
$F_{y\Phi LP}$	Resulting $F_{y\Phi}$ signals after low-pass filter
$F_{y\Phi CAD}$	Cadence signals obtained from the FLC
M	Order of the FLC filter
μ	Adaptive gain of the FLC filter
F	Final force applied to the walker by the user
τ	Final torque applied to the walker by the user
$F_{yLeftLP}$	Resulting signal from the low-pass filter for F_{yLeft}
$F_{yLeftCAD}$	Resulting signal from the FLC for F_{yLeft}
v	Linear velocity generated with an admittance controller
ω	Angular velocity generated with an admittance controller
$L(s)$	Second order system for linear velocities generation
m	Virtual mass of the walker
b_l	Damping ratio for $L(s)$
k_l	Elastic constant for $L(s)$
$A(s)$	Second order system for angular velocities generation

J	Virtual moment of inertia of the walker
b_a	Damping ratio for $A(s)$
k_a	Elastic constant for $A(s)$
SLAM	Simultaneous Localization and Mapping
AMCL	Adaptive Monte Carlo Localization Approach
TEB	Time Elastic Band
ROI	Region of interest in the camera image
HOG	Histogram of Oriented Gradients
SVM	Support Vector Machine
STD	Stop Distance Parameter
SD	Slow Distance Parameter
WR	Width Rate
MET	Maximum Exerted Torque
$x_n av$	X position of nearest path point
$y_n av$	Y position of nearest path point
$x_s w$	X position of the walker
$y_n av$	Y position of the walker
θ_{sw}	Orientation of the walker
θ_{usr}	Orientation of user's intention of movement
θ_{nav}	Orientation of nearest path point
d	Euclidean distance from the walker position to the next pose
La	Base of first right-angled triangle
Lb	Base of second right-angled triangle
θ_a	Auxiliary angle for first right-angled triangle
θ_b	Auxiliary angle for first right-angled triangle
Win_{width}	Scaling factor of triangle-shaped window
θ_{nxt}	Orientation of next path pose
θ_{diff}	Relative orientation of the triangle-shaped window center

References

1. Buchman, A.S.; Boyle, P.A.; Leurgans, S.E.; Barnes, L.L.; Bennett, D.A. Cognitive Function is Associated with the Development of Mobility Impairments in Community-Dwelling Elders. *Am. J. Geriatr. Psychiatry* **2011**, *19*, 571–580. [CrossRef] [PubMed]
2. Pirker, W.; Katzenschlager, R. Gait disorders in adults and the elderly. *Wien. Klin. Wochenschr.* **2017**, *129*, 81–95. [CrossRef] [PubMed]
3. Mrozowski, J.; Awrejcewicz, J.; Bamberski, P. Analysis of stability of the human gait. *J. Theor. Appl. Mech.* **2007**, *45*, 91–98.
4. Cifuentes, C.A.; Frizera, A. *Human-Robot Interaction Strategies for Walker-Assisted Locomotion; Springer Tracts in Advanced Robotics*; Springer: Cham, Switzerland, 2016; Volume 115, p. 105. [CrossRef]
5. Mikolajczyk, T.; Ciobanu, I.; Badea, D.I.; Iliescu, A.; Pizzamiglio, S.; Schauer, T.; Seel, T.; Seiciu, P.L.; Turner, D.L.; Berteanu, M. Advanced technology for gait rehabilitation: An overview. *Adv. Mech. Eng.* **2018**, *10*, 1–19. [CrossRef]
6. Gheno, R.; Cepparo, J.M.; Rosca, C.E.; Cotten, A. Musculoskeletal Disorders in the Elderly. *J. Clin. Imaging Sci.* **2012**, *2*, 39. [CrossRef]
7. World Health Organization. Disability and Health. 2018. Available online: https://www.who.int/news-room/fact-sheets/detail/disability-and-health (accessed on 29 June 2019).
8. World Health Organization. *World Report on Disability 2011*; World Health Organization: Geneva, Switzerland, 2011.
9. World Health Organization. *Ageing and Health*; World Health Organization: Geneva, Switzerland, 2018.
10. The World Bank. Disability Inclusion. 2018. Available online: https://www.worldbank.org/en/topic/disability (accessed on 29 June 2019).

11. Pedersen, M.M.; Holt, N.E.; Grande, L.; Kurlinski, L.A.; Beauchamp, M.K.; Kiely, D.K.; Petersen, J.; Leveille, S.; Bean, J.F. Mild cognitive impairment status and mobility performance: An analysis from the Boston RISE study. *J. Gerontol. Ser. Biol. Sci. Med. Sci.* **2014**, *69*, 1511–1518. [CrossRef]
12. Brown, C.J.; Flood, K.L. Mobility limitation in the older patient: A clinical review. *JAMA J. Am. Med. Assoc.* **2013**, *310*, 1168–1177. [CrossRef]
13. Chaparro-Cárdenas, S.L.; Lozano-Guzmán, A.A.; Ramirez-Bautista, J.A.; Hernández-Zavala, A. A review in gait rehabilitation devices and applied control techniques. *Disabil. Rehabil. Assist. Technol.* **2018**, [CrossRef]
14. Martins, M.M.; Frizera-Neto, A.; Urendes, E.; dos Santos, C.; Ceres, R.; Bastos-Filho, T. A novel human-machine interface for guiding: The NeoASAS smart walker. In Proceedings of the IEEE 2012 ISSNIP Biosignals and Biorobotics Conference: Biosignals and Robotics for Better and Safer Living (BRC), Manaus, Brazil, 9–11 January 2012; pp. 1–7. [CrossRef]
15. Bateni, H.; Maki, B.E. Assistive devices for balance and mobility: Benefits, demands, and adverse consequences. *Arch. Phys. Med. Rehabil.* **2005**, *86*, 134–145. [CrossRef]
16. Neto, A.F.; Elias, A.; Cifuentes, C.; Rodriguez, C.; Bastos, T.; Carelli, R. Smart Walkers: Advanced Robotic Human Walking-Aid Systems. In *Springer Tracts in Advanced Robotics 106 Intelligent Assistive Robots Recent Advances in Assistive Robotics*; Springer: Cham, Switzerland, 2015; pp. 103–131. [CrossRef]
17. Geravand, M.; Werner, C.; Hauer, K.; Peer, A. An Integrated Decision Making Approach for Adaptive Shared Control of Mobility Assistance Robots. *Int. J. Soc. Robot.* **2016**, *8*, 631–648. [CrossRef]
18. Mitzner, T.L.; Chen, T.L.; Kemp, C.C.; Rogers, W.A. Identifying the Potential for Robotics to Assist Older Adults in Different Living Environments. *Int. J. Soc. Robot.* **2014**, *6*, 213–227. [CrossRef] [PubMed]
19. Jenkins, S.; Draper, H. Care, Monitoring, and Companionship: Views on Care Robots from Older People and Their Carers. *Int. J. Soc. Robot.* **2015**, *7*, 673–683. [CrossRef]
20. Martins, M.; Santos, C.; Frizera, A.; Ceres, R. A review of the functionalities of smart walkers. *Med. Eng. Phys.* **2015**, *37*, 917–928. [CrossRef] [PubMed]
21. Martins, M.; Santos, C.; Seabra, E.; Frizera, A.; Ceres, R. Design, implementation and testing of a new user interface for a smart walker. In Proceedings of the 2014 IEEE International Conference on Autonomous Robot Systems and Competitions (ICARSC), Espinho, Portugal, 14–15 May 2014; pp. 217–222. [CrossRef]
22. Lacey, G.J.; Rodriguez-Losada, D. The evolution of guido. *IEEE Robot. Autom. Mag.* **2008**, *15*, 75–83. [CrossRef]
23. Morris, A.; Donamukkala, R.; Kapuria, A.; Steinfeld, A.; Matthews, J.; Dunbar-Jacob, J.; Thrun, S. A robotic walker that provides guidance. In Proceedings of the 2003 IEEE International Conference on Robotics and Automation (Cat. No. 03CH37422), Taipei, Taiwan, 14–19 September 2003; Volume 1, pp. 25–30. [CrossRef]
24. Alves, J.; Seabra, E.; Caetano, I.; Santos, C.P. Overview of the ASBGo++ Smart Walker. In Proceedings of the 2017 IEEE 5th Portuguese Meeting on Bioengineering (ENBENG), Coimbra, Portugal, 16–18 February 2017; pp. 1–4. [CrossRef]
25. Caetano, I.; Alves, J.; Goncalves, J.; Martins, M.; Santos, C.P. Development of a Biofeedback Approach Using Body Tracking with Active Depth Sensor in ASBGo Smart Walker. In Proceedings of the 2016 International Conference on Autonomous Robot Systems and Competitions (ICARSC), Bragança, Portugal, 4–6 May 2016; pp. 241–246. [CrossRef]
26. Lee, G.; Ohnuma, T.; Chong, N.Y. Design and control of JAIST active robotic walker. *Intell. Serv. Robot.* **2010**, *3*, 125–135. [CrossRef]
27. Lee, G.; Jung, E.J.; Ohnuma, T.; Chong, N.Y.; Yi, B.J. JAIST Robotic Walker control based on a two-layered Kalman filter. In Proceedings of the IEEE International Conference on Robotics and Automation, Shanghai, China, 9–13 May 2011; pp. 3682–3687. [CrossRef]
28. Jiménez, M.F.; Monllor, M.; Frizera, A.; Bastos, T.; Roberti, F.; Carelli, R. Admittance Controller with Spatial Modulation for Assisted Locomotion using a Smart Walker. *J. Intell. Robot. Syst.* **2019**, *94*, 621–637. [CrossRef]
29. Spenko, M.; Yu, H.; Dubowsky, S. Robotic personal aids for mobility and monitoring for the elderly. *IEEE Trans. Neural Syst. Rehabil. Eng.* **2006**, *14*, 344–351. [CrossRef]
30. Efthimiou, E.; Fotinea, S.E.; Goulas, T.; Dimou, A.L.; Koutsombogera, M.; Pitsikalis, V.; Maragos, P.; Tzafestas, C. *The MOBOT Platform—Showcasing Multimodality in Human-Assistive Robot Interaction*; Springer: Cham, Switzerland, 2016; pp. 382–391. [CrossRef]

31. Efthimiou, E.; Fotinea, S.E.; Goulas, T.; Koutsombogera, M.; Karioris, P.; Vacalopoulou, A.; Rodomagoulakis, I.; Maragos, P.; Tzafestas, C.; Pitsikalis, V.; et al. The MOBOT rollator human-robot interaction model and user evaluation process. In Proceedings of the 2016 IEEE Symposium Series on Computational Intelligence (SSCI 2016), Athens, Greece, 6–9 December 2019. [CrossRef]
32. Papageorgiou, X.S.; Chalvatzaki, G.; Lianos, K.N.; Werner, C.; Hauer, K.; Tzafestas, C.S.; Maragos, P. Experimental validation of human pathological gait analysis for an assisted living intelligent robotic walker. In Proceedings of the IEEE RAS and EMBS International Conference on Biomedical Robotics and Biomechatronics, Pisa, Italy, 20–22 February 2016; pp. 1086–1091. [CrossRef]
33. Mou, W.H.; Chang, M.F.; Liao, C.K.; Hsu, Y.H.; Tseng, S.H.; Fu, L.C. Context-aware assisted interactive robotic walker for Parkinson's disease patients. In Proceedings of the 2012 IEEE/RSJ International Conference on Intelligent Robots and Systems, Vilamoura, Portugal, 7–12 October 2012; pp. 329–334. [CrossRef]
34. Paulo, J.; Peixoto, P.; Nunes, U.J. ISR-AIWALKER: Robotic Walker for Intuitive and Safe Mobility Assistance and Gait Analysis. *IEEE Trans. Hum. Mach. Syst.* **2017**, *47*, 1110–1122. [CrossRef]
35. Garrote, L.; Paulo, J.; Perdiz, J.; Peixoto, P.; Nunes, U.J. Robot-Assisted Navigation for a Robotic Walker with Aided User Intent. In Proceedings of the RO-MAN 2018—27th IEEE International Symposium on Robot and Human Interactive Communication, Nanjing, China, 27 August–1 September 2018; pp. 348–355. [CrossRef]
36. Huang, C.; Wasson, G.; Alwan, M.; Sheth, P. Shared Navigational Control and User Intent Detection in an Intelligent Walker. 2005. Available online: https://www.aaai.org/Papers/Symposia/Fall/2005/FS-05-02/FS05-02-010.pdf (accessed on 29 June 2019).
37. Wachaja, A.; Agarwal, P.; Zink, M.; Adame, M.R.; Möller, K.; Burgard, W. Navigating blind people with walking impairments using a smart walker. *Auton. Robot.* **2017**, *41*, 555–573. [CrossRef]
38. Wasson, G.; Gunderson, J.; Graves, S.; Felder, R. Effective Shared Control in Cooperative Mobility Aids. In Proceedings of the Fourteenth international Florida Artificial intelligence Research Society Conference, Key West, FL, USA, 21–23 May 2001; AAAI Press: Menlo Park, CA, USA, 2001; pp. 509–513.
39. Wasson, G.; Gunderson, J.; Graves, S.; Felder, R. An assistive robotic agent for pedestrian mobility. In Proceedings of the Fifth International Conference on Autonomous Agents—AGENTS'01, Montreal, QC, Canada, 28 May–1 June 2001; ACM Press: New York, NY, USA, 2001; pp. 169–173. [CrossRef]
40. Palopoli, L.; Argyros, A.; Birchbauer, J.; Colombo, A.; Fontanelli, D.; Legay, A.; Garulli, A.; Giannitrapani, A.; Macii, D.; Moro, F.; et al. Navigation assistance and guidance of older adults across complex public spaces: The DALi approach. *Intell. Serv. Robot.* **2015**, *8*, 77–92. [CrossRef]
41. Cheng, W.C.; Wu, Y.Z. A user's intention detection method for smart walker. In Proceedings of the 2017 IEEE 8th International Conference on Awareness Science and Technology (iCAST), Taiwan, China, 8–10 November 2017; pp. 35–39. [CrossRef]
42. Ye, J.; Huang, J.; He, J.; Tao, C.; Wang, X. Development of a width-changeable intelligent walking-aid robot. In Proceedings of the 2012 International Symposium on Micro-NanoMechatronics and Human Science (MHS), Nagoya, Japan, 4–7 November 2012; pp. 358–363. [CrossRef]
43. Hirata, Y.; Hara, A.; Kosuge, K. Passive-type intelligent walking support system "RT Walker". In Proceedings of the 2004 IEEE/RSJ International Conference on Intelligent Robots and Systems (IROS) (IEEE Cat. No. 04CH37566), Sendai, Japan, 28 September–2 October 2004; Volume 4, pp. 3871–3876. [CrossRef]
44. Frizera-Neto, A.; Ceres, R.; Rocon, E.; Pons, J.L. Empowering and assisting natural human mobility: The simbiosis walker. *Int. J. Adv. Robot. Syst.* **2011**, *8*, 34–50. [CrossRef]
45. Kulyukin, V.; Kutiyanawala, A.; LoPresti, E.; Matthews, J.; Simpson, R. IWalker: Toward a rollator-mounted wayfinding system for the elderly. In Proceedings of the 2008 IEEE International Conference on RFID (Frequency Identification), Amman, Jordan, 20–22 July 2008; pp. 303–311.
46. Lu, C.K.; Huang, Y.C.; Lee, C.J. Adaptive guidance system design for the assistive robotic walker. *Neurocomputing* **2015**, *170*, 152–160. [CrossRef]
47. Reyes Adame, M.; Yu, J.; Moeller, K. Mobility Support System for Elderly Blind People with a Smart Walker and a Tactile Map. *IFMBE Proc.* **2016**, *57*, 602–607. [CrossRef]
48. Thorstensson, A.; Nilsson, J.; Carlson, H.; Zomlefer, M.R. Trunk movements in human locomotion. *Acta Physiol. Scand.* **1984**, *121*, 9–22. [CrossRef] [PubMed]

49. Bonnet, V.; Mazzà, C.; McCamley, J.; Cappozzo, A. Use of weighted Fourier linear combiner filters to estimate lower trunk 3D orientation from gyroscope sensors data. *J. Neuroeng. Rehabil.* **2013**, *10*, 29. [CrossRef] [PubMed]
50. Neto, A.F.; Gallego, J.A.; Rocon, E.; Abellanas, A.; Pons, J.L.; Ceres, R. Online Cadence Estimation through Force Interaction in Walker Assisted Gait. In Proceedings of the ISSNIP Biosignals and Biorobotics Conference 2010, Vitoria, Brazil, 4–6 January 2010; pp. 1–5.
51. Frizera Neto, A.; Gallego, J.A.; Rocon, E.; Pons, J.L.; Ceres, R. Extraction of user's navigation commands from upper body force interaction in walker assisted gait. *BioMed. Eng. Online* **2010**, *9*, 1–16. [CrossRef] [PubMed]
52. Sierra, S.D.; Molina, J.F.; Gómez, D.A.; Cifuentes, C.A.; Múnera, M.C. Development of an Interface for Human-Robot Interaction on a Robotic Platform for Gait Assistance: AGoRA Smart Walker. In Proceedings of the 2018 IEEE ANDESCON, Santiago de Cali, Colombia, 22–24 August 2018.
53. Grisetti, G.; Stachniss, C.; Burgard, W. Improved Techniques for Grid Mapping With Rao-Blackwellized Particle Filters. *IEEE Trans. Robot.* **2007**, *23*, 34–46. [CrossRef]
54. Fox, D.; Burgard, W.; Dellaert, F.; Thrun, S. Monte Carlo Localization: Efficient Position Estimation for Mobile Robots. In Proceedings of the Sixteenth National Conference on Artificial Intelligence and Eleventh Conference on Innovative Applications of Artificial Intelligence, Orlando, FL, USA, 8–22 July 1999; pp. 343–349.
55. Lu, D.V.; Hershberger, D.; Smart, W.D. Layered costmaps for context-sensitive navigation. In Proceedings of the 2014 IEEE/RSJ International Conference on Intelligent Robots and Systems, Chicago, IL, USA, 14–18 September 2014; pp. 709–715. [CrossRef]
56. Fox, D.; Burgard, W.; Thrun, S. The Dynamic Window Approach to Collision Avoidance. *Robot. Autom. Mag.* **1997**, *4*, 1–23. [CrossRef]
57. Rösmann, C.; Feiten, W.; Wösch, T.; Hoffmann, F.; Bertram, T. Trajectory modification considering dynamic constraints of autonomous robots. In Proceedings of the 7th German Conference on Robotics, Munich, Germany, 21–22 May 2012; pp. 74–79.
58. Fotiadis, E.P.; Garzón, M.; Barrientos, A. Human detection from a mobile robot using fusion of laser and vision information. *Sensors* **2013**, *13*, 11603–11635. [CrossRef]
59. Garzon Oviedo, M.A.; Barrientos, A.; Del Cerro, J.; Alacid, A.; Fotiadis, E.; Rodríguez-Canosa, G.R.; Wang, B.C. Tracking and following pedestrian trajectories, an approach for autonomous surveillance of critical infrastructures. *Ind. Robot. Int. J.* **2015**, *42*, 429–440. [CrossRef]
60. Arras, K.O.; Lau, B.; Grzonka, S.; Luber, M.; Mozos, O.M.; Meyer-Delius, D.; Burgard, W. Range-Based People Detection and Tracking for Socially Enabled Service Robots. In *Towards Service Robots for Everyday Environments*; Springer Tracts in Advanced Robotics; Springer: Berlin/Heidelberg, Germany, 2012; Volume 76, pp. 235–280. [CrossRef]
61. Schapire, R.E.; Schapire, R.E. Improved Boosting Algorithms Using Confidence-rated Predictions. *Computer* **1999**, *336*, 297–336. [CrossRef]
62. Zhang, Q.; Pless, R. Extrinsic Calibration of a Camera and Laser Range Finder (improves camera calibration). *IROS* **2004**, *3*, 2301–2306. [CrossRef]
63. Dalal, N.; Triggs, B. Histograms of oriented gradients for human detection. In Proceedings of the 2005 IEEE Computer Society Conference on Computer Vision and Pattern Recognition (CVPR 2005), San Diego, CA, USA, 20–25 June 2005; Volume I, pp. 886–893. [CrossRef]
64. Niculescu-Mizil, A.; Caruana, R. Predicting good probabilities with supervised learning. In Proceedings of the 22nd International Conference on Machine Learning (ICML'05), Bonn, Germany, 7–11 August 2005; pp. 625–632. [CrossRef]
65. Papadakis, P.; Rives, P.; Spalanzani, A. Adaptive spacing in human-robot interactions. In Proceedings of the 2014 IEEE/RSJ International Conference on Intelligent Robots and Systems, Chicago, IL, USA, 14–18 September 2014; pp. 2627–2632. [CrossRef]
66. Venkatesh, V.; Morris, M.G.; Davis, G.B.; Davis, F.D. User Acceptance of Information Technology: Toward a Unified View. *MIS Q.* **2003**, *27*, 425. [CrossRef]
67. Venkatesh, V.; Thong, J.Y.L.; Xu, X. Consumer Acceptance and Use of Information Technology: Extending the Unified Theory. *MIS Q.* **2012**, *36*, 157–178. [CrossRef]

68. Joost, C.F.; Dodou, D. Five-Point Likert Items: t test versus Mann-Whitney-Wilcoxon. *Pract. Assess. Res. Eval.* **2010**, *15*, 1–16.
69. Blair, R.C.; Higgins, J.J. A Comparison of the Power of Wilcoxon's Rank-Sum Statistic to That of Student's t Statistic under Various Nonnormal Distributions. *J. Educ. Stat.* **1980**, *5*, 309. [CrossRef]

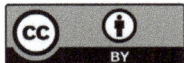

© 2019 by the authors. Licensee MDPI, Basel, Switzerland. This article is an open access article distributed under the terms and conditions of the Creative Commons Attribution (CC BY) license (http://creativecommons.org/licenses/by/4.0/).

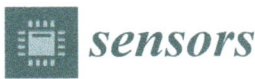

Article

Physiological Responses During Hybrid BNCI Control of an Upper-Limb Exoskeleton

Francisco J. Badesa [1,2,8,*], Jorge A. Diez [1,8,*], Jose Maria Catalan [1,8], Emilio Trigili [3], Francesca Cordella [5], Marius Nann [6], Simona Crea [3,7,9], Surjo R. Soekadar [4], Loredana Zollo [5], Nicola Vitiello [3,7,9], Nicolas Garcia-Aracil [1,8]

1. Miguel Hernández University of Elche, Av. Universidad w/n, Ed. Innova, 03202 Alicante, Spain; jcatalan@umh.es (J.M.C.); nicolas.garcia@umh.es (N.G.-A.)
2. Universidad de Cádiz, Av. de la Universidad n10, 11519 Puerto Real, Spain
3. The BioRobotics Institute, Scuola Superiore Sant'Anna, Viale Rinaldo Piaggio 34, 56025 Pontedera, Pisa, Italy; e.trigili@santannapisa.it (E.T.); s.crea@santannapisa.it (S.C.); nicola.vitiello@santannapisa.it (N.V.)
4. Clinical Neurotechnology Laboratory, Department of Psychiatry and Psychotherapy (CCM), Charité-Universitätsmedizin Berlin, Charitéplatz 1, 10117 Berlin, Germany; surjo.soekadar@charite.de
5. Unit of Advanced Robotics and Human-centred Technologies, Campus Bio-Medico University of Rome, 00128 Rome, Italy; f.cordella@unicampus.it (F.C.); L.Zollo@unicampus.it (L.Z.)
6. Applied Neurotechnology Laboratory, Department of Psychiatry and Psychotherapy, University Hopsital of Tübingen, Calwerstr. 14, 72076 Tübingen, Germany; marius.nann@uni-tuebingen.de
7. IRCCS Fondazione Don Carlo Gnocchi, Via Alfonso Capecelatro 66, 20148 Milan, Italy
8. New technologies for Neurorehabilitation Lab., Av. de la Hospitalidad, s/n, 28054 Madrid, Spain
9. Department of Excellence in Robotics & AI, Scuola Superiore Sant'Anna, 56025 Pontedera, Pisa, Italy
* Correspondence: javier.badesa@uca.es (F.J.B.); jdiez@umh.es (J.A.D.)

Received: 30 September 2019; Accepted: 5 November 2019; Published: 12 November 2019

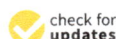

Abstract: When combined with assistive robotic devices, such as wearable robotics, brain/neural-computer interfaces (BNCI) have the potential to restore the capabilities of handicapped people to carry out activities of daily living. To improve applicability of such systems, workload and stress should be reduced to a minimal level. Here, we investigated the user's physiological reactions during the exhaustive use of the interfaces of a hybrid control interface. Eleven BNCI-naive healthy volunteers participated in the experiments. All participants sat in a comfortable chair in front of a desk and wore a whole-arm exoskeleton as well as wearable devices for monitoring physiological, electroencephalographic (EEG) and electrooculographic (EoG) signals. The experimental protocol consisted of three phases: (i) Set-up, calibration and BNCI training; (ii) Familiarization phase ; and (iii) Experimental phase during which each subject had to perform EEG and EoG tasks. After completing each task, the NASA-TLX questionnaire and self-assessment manikin (SAM) were completed by the user. We found significant differences (p-value < 0.05) in heart rate variability (HRV) and skin conductance level (SCL) between participants during the use of the two different biosignal modalities (EEG, EoG) of the BNCI. This indicates that EEG control is associated with a higher level of stress (associated with a decrease in HRV) and mental work load (associated with a higher level of SCL) when compared to EoG control. In addition, HRV and SCL modulations correlated with the subject's workload perception and emotional responses assessed through NASA-TLX questionnaires and SAM.

Keywords: Assistive technologies; exoskeleton; brain-computer interfaces

1. Introduction

Around 80 million people in the EU, a sixth of its population, have a disability. They are often hindered from full social and economic participation by various barriers related to physical, psychological and social factors. Over 30% of people above the age of 75 are impaired to some extent, and over 20% are severely impaired. The percentage of people with disabilities is set to rise as the EU population ages [1].

Using brain-machine interfaces (BMIs) or brain-computer interfaces (BCIs) in combination with assistive robotic devices, such as wearable robots, has the potential to augment the capabilities of disabled people to carry out activities of daily living with success. Recent developments of BMIs or BCIs allow detection and translation of electric, magnetic or metabolic activity into control signals of external devices or machines. However, reliability and safety of these systems are insufficient for daily life applications. Thus, fusion of different bio-signals under the concept of brain/neural-computer interaction (BNCI) systems, also referred as hybrid BCIs or multimodal BCIs. They were introduced for the first time by [2].

The different BNCI approaches can be distinguished accordingly with the type of bio-signals used as inputs in the control of assistive or rehabilitation devices [3]. The first approach is based on the combination of different brain signals, such as Event-related Potential (ERP) and sensorimotor rhythm (SMR) induced by Motor Imagery (MI) [4], ERP and Steady State Evoked Potential (SSEP) [5–7], and SMR and SSEP [8,9]. The second approach is based on the fusion or combination of brain signals and other kind of bio-signals, such as sEMG [10,11], ECG [12,13] and electrooculography (EoG) [14,15].

On the other hand, there are already published some examples of multi-modal architectures for the interaction and control of upper-limb robotic exoskeletons. Specifically, Frisoli et al. presented a robotic-assisted rehabilitation training with an upper limb robotic exoskeleton for the restoration of motor function in spatial reaching movements [16]. Then, they presented a multimodal control of an arm-hand robotic exoskeleton to perform activities of daily living. The presented system was driven by a shared control architecture using BCI and eye gaze tracking for the control of an arm exoskeleton and a hand exoskeleton for reaching and grasping/releasing cylindrical objects of different size in the framework of the BRAVO project [17]. Moreover, Pedrocchi et al. developed a novel system composed by a passive arm exoskeleton, robotic hand orthosis and a neuro muscular electrical stimulation system driven by residual voluntary muscular activation, head/eye motion, and brain signals in the framework of the MUNDUS project [18].

Differently from the previous works, the multimodal approach, developed inside the AIDE European project, is based on a hybrid control interface based on the combination of a gaze tracking, electroencephalography (EEG) and EoG system to intuitively control an arm/hand exoskeleton for assisting in reaching and grasping objects to people with disabilities (see Figure 1). The AIDE multimodal control interface predicts the activity user wants to perform and allows the user to trigger the execution of different sub-actions that compose the predicted activity, and to interrupt the task at any time by means of the hybrid control interface.

The user's psychological state is related to the use and performance in brain-computer interface seems to be a well accepted statement, but there are not so many studies to corroborate it. Kaufmann et al. in [19] studied correlations between P300-BCI based task performance and resting heart rate variability, reporting that frequency domain measures of heart rate variability were significantly associated with BCI-performance. Moreover, the correlation between the use BCI and fatigue, frustration and attention were investigated in [20,21], indicating that mental state was closely related to BCI use and performance; in [22],discriminating four levels of attention which can be used for boosting the BCI performance;and in [23], classifying three attention levels using a KNN classifier based on the Self-Assessment Manikin (SAM) model.

There are currently two use scenarios for BNCI systems: brain/neural control of assistive devices, such as wearable robots and prostheses, and use of BNCI systems for rehabilitation [24,25]. In the context of the first use scenario, involving EEG-signals, typically related to imagined or attempted actions, offers the advantage of intuitive control. Here, combination with EOG signals can improve real-world applicability of brain controlled devices, because EOG control is very accessible and can provide a reliable veto-function [26]. At the same time, EEG control can be cumbersome, particularly when the classification accuracy is rather low (e.g., due to low signal quality/artefacts) or when the user has not yet gained stable BNCI control. In the context of the second scenario, in contrast, brain signals are used to induce neuroplasticity triggering neural recovery [25]. Recently, it was suggested to combine both approaches, the assistive and restorative approach, to increase user acceptability and broad adoption of BNCI-based rehabilitation [27]. For this purpose, EEG/EOG brain/neural control has to be optimized in terms of mental work load and user engagement accessible through the subject's physiological responses. Assessment of physiological responses during EEG/EOG brain/neural control would not only allow for designing optimal control strategies, but may also inform adaptation of the BNCI system during actual use (e.g., by providing feedback about the optimal window of operation, adapting the bio-signal detection thresholds etc.). In this paper, the user's physiological reactions related to an exhaustive use of the interfaces in the brain/neural control of an assistive wearable arm/hand exoskeleton is analysed in two ways: in terms of the evolution and changes during a specific task; and the differences between the use of two different interfaces (EEG and EoG).

2. Materials and Methods

2.1. Multimodal Sensory System

All participants were sitting in a conformable chair in front of a desk and wore a whole-arm exoskeleton as well as wearable devices for monitoring physiological, EEG and EoG signals (Figure 1).

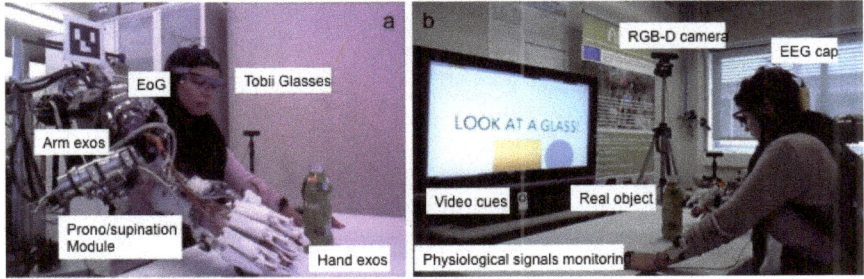

Figure 1. Experimental setup: All the assistive technology shown in the figure was developed in the AIDE EU project framework to assist arm and hand function after severe paralysis. (**a**): Wearable eye tracker (Tobbi Glasses), electrooculography (EoG) interface, arm exoskeleton including pronosupination module and hand exoskelton. (**b**): A context-sensitive 3D-camera and visual feedback support precise and reliable assistance to grasp a real object; EEG and physiological signals monitoring system.

2.1.1. Hybrid Bnci

The hybrid BNCI interface was used to control a vision-guided autonomous whole-arm exoskeleton to perform reaching and grassping tasks. The shared-human control of the whole-arm exoskeleton was implemented using a finite-state machine (FSM) triggered by electroencephalography/electrooculography (EEG/EOG) signals similar to the presented in [28]. Specifically, the reaching task was controlled by an EOG signal related to horizontal oculoversions (HOV) to the right (HOVr) and the hand closing task was controlled by computing the user intention through motor imagery-related EEG desynchronization of sensorimotor rhythms (SMR-ERD also termed μ-rhythm; 8 to 15 Hz) [26]. The SMR-ERD was computed using the power method proposed by Pfurtscheller and Lopes da Silva [29]. The EEG/EOG singals were recorded using the Enobio 8 (Neuroelectrics, Barcelona, Spain), an eight-channel wireless EEG recording system. The EEG signals were recorded from 5 electrodes placed at F3, T3, C3, Cz and P3 locations according to the 10–20 international system with ground and reference electrodes at AFz and FCz respectively. The last channel of Enobio system was used to detect the voluntary horizontal oculoversions (HOV) using EoG signals recorded from the left outer canthus referenced to left mastoid. Instead of conventional electrolyte gel electrodes, polyamide-based dry electrodes were used [30]. These electrodes might be a viable solution to substantially improve the cost-benefit ratio of wearing comfort, preparation time, user-friendliness, long-term stability, reliability and financial costs. EEG signals was recorded at a sampling rate of 200 Hz, band-pass filtered at 0.4–70 Hz and pre-processed using a Hjorth Laplacian filter centered on C3 electrode to attenuate line noise and movement artefacts [31]. Similar to EEG signal processing, EOG signals was recorded at a sampling rate of 200 Hz and pre-processed using a band-pass filtered at 0.1–30 Hz. A customized version of the open-source BCI2000 were used to calibrate and to translate user's biosignals into control signals of the vision-guided autonomous whole-arm exoskeleton [26]. During the calibration, the following key features were computed: (i) the reference value (RV) of SMR-ERD related to externally paced intended grasping movements; (ii) the optimal frequency for SMR-ERD detection; (iii) the SMR-ED detection threshold; and (iv) the HOV detection threshold (Figure 2).

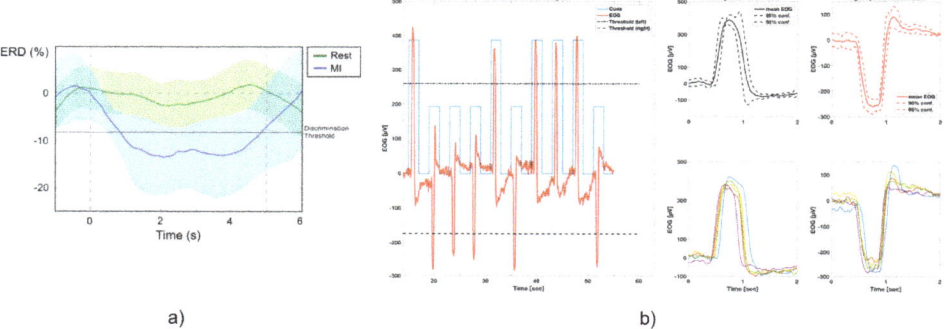

Figure 2. (Example of ERD and EOG control signals. (**a**) Example of event-related desynchronization (ERD) of "rest" and "motor imagery" (MI) phase. During calibration, discrimination threshold for reliable differentiation is set. (**b**) Overview of EOG control signals. Left side: EOG time series of horizontal eye movements (red). Movements are cued to left (blue long bars) and right (blue short bars) movements. Black dotted lines represent 60% discrimination thresholds based on maximum EOG peaks. Right side: Time-locked EOG signals of left/right horizontal eye movements during cue presentations. Plots show mean EOG with 95% confidence intervals (upper figures), which is calculated out of the EOG raw signals (lower figures).

2.1.2. Physiological Monitoring System

The physiological monitoring system acquires and processes signals, such as, electrocardiography (ECG), galvanic skin response (GSR) and respiratory plethysmography.

The selection of components of the sensory system for the physiological monitoring system was based on the requirements imposed by its application to the robotic assistance in daily life activities. Therefore, all devices need to be wearable and wireless, preferably directly on-body with combined sensor, processing and sending unit not to disturb users through connection or power cables during daily life tasks.

BioHarness 3 and Shimmer 3 GSR+ Unit, are wearable, wireless and provide a high wearing comfort to monitor ECG, respiratory plethysmography and GSR. Both devices have a built-in signal-processing unit sending the resulting information to the main processing unit via Bluetooth where further processing is performed.

The BioHarness 3 is a compact physiological monitoring device developed by Zephyr Technology. The device is based on a wearable strap that is placed around the chest. The strap contains the actual physiological sensors and a computing unit with Bluetooth module. Supported recording techniques are ECG, respiratory plethysmographie, skin temperature and acceleration measurement. This means that the BioHarness 3 can output the requested heart rate (HR), respiration rate (RR) and heart rate variability (HRV) which is a measure of the variation in time between each heartbeat. In particular, the SDANN is used as a feature of HRV, which is defined as the standard deviation of the average instantaneous heart rate intervals (NN) calculated over short periods. In our case, the SDANN is computed over a moving window of 300 s.

The Shimmer3 GSR+ Unit measures skin conductivity between two reusable electrodes mounted to two fingers of one hand. The output measure is the galvanic skin response (GSR). GSR is a common measure in psychophysiological paradigms and therefore often used in affective state detection.

2.2. Arm Exoskeleton

The arm exoskeleton can be splitted into two main parts: (i) a hand-wrist exoskeleton; and (ii) a shoulder-elbow exoskeleton.

2.2.1. Shoulder-Elbow Exoskeleton

The shoulder-elbow exoskeleton (NESM) has four active degrees of freedom, namely shoulder adduction/abduction, flexion/extension and intra/extra rotation and elbow flexion/extension, together with eight additional passive degrees of freedom for the alignment of the motor axes to the human joint axes, regardless the user's specific anthropometry sizes [32,33].

The main novelty introduced by this system relies on its mechanical architecture: the actuation units of the NESM are based on a Series Elastic Actuation (SEA) architecture. SEAs reduce the mechanical stiffness of the actuator and are easy to control in position mode and torque modes. Moreover, simple software algorithms can be implemented to monitor the torque delivered at each joint and avoid exceeding specific values, as well as detecting collisions with external objects.

2.2.2. Hand-Wrist Exoskeleton

The hand-wrist exoskeleton is composed of two modules, the hand and the wrist, that can be used separately or in combination. The hand exoskeleton has three active degrees-of-freedom, corresponding to flexion-extension of index finger, flexion-extension of middle finger and flexion-extension of both ring and little finger. The thumb will have a series of passive-degrees of freedom that will allow placing the thumb in a suitable pose in the installation phase, and will be lockable to allow the thumb to work in opposition during the grasp [34].

The wrist exoskeleton was designed to be easily connected to the NESM exoskeleton.

2.3. Participants

Eleven BNCI-naive volunteers participated in the experiments(six males and five females). None of the study participants had any prior experience in the use of these kind of interfaces. All were healthy, without cognitive or physical deficits. They were aged between 26 and 42 (mean age 31 years, median age 29 years, standard deviation 6.3 years). Before inclusion, participants gave their written informed consent, including photography and video, and agreed that this material can be used in journals and other public media. The study protocol was approved by the local ethics committee of the Miguel Hernandez University (Elche, Spain).

2.4. Experimental Protocol

The experimental protocol consists of three phases:

1. **Set-up, calibration and BNCI training:** Calibration of the BNCI system comprises two parts: in the first part, participants are instructed to either relax or imagine hand-grasping motions following a visual cue displayed on a computer screen. To identify the optimal frequency for detection of motor-imagery related desynchronization of sensorimotor rhythms (SMR, 8–15Hz) of the subject, a power spectrum estimation is performed, selecting the frequency that shows largest

even-related desynchronization (ERD) during motor-imagery and event-related synchronization (ERS) during relax. Based on the maximum values for ERD and ERS, an optimal discrimination threshold is computed and used for later online BCI control. EoG is recorded in accordance to the standard EoG placements at the left and right outer canthus (LOC/ROC). In the EoG-related part of the calibration, subjects are instructed to move their eyes to the left or to the right following randomized visual cues (arrow to the left, arrow to the right). A detection threshold for full left and right eye movements is set at 80% of the average of maximal EoG signal recorded during presentation of the visual cues.

2. **Familiarization:** The familiarization phase only consisted of showing the user the functioning of the finite-state machine and the visual interface. No additional training was required, since the user was already familiarized with the EEG/EoG interface.

3. **Experimental phase:** Each subject had to perform two different tasks during 6 min each one: (i) a task triggered by the EoG interface to reach an object controlling the arm exoskeleton; (ii) a task triggered by the EEG interface to grasp an object controlling the hand exoskeleton. To increase the number of data points for the analysis, subjects were asked to perform two times the EoG task and four times the EEG task. After completing each task with one interface, the NASA-TLX questionnaire and self-assessment manikin (SAM) were submitted to the user to evaluate the subjective workload required to perform the task.

3. Results

For each participant, both objective and subjective measurements were analysed and quantified. For objective values, some parameters were computed: (i) the performance using each interface; (ii) the activation time computed as the average time to trigger each movement with each interface; and (iii) features extracted from the analysis of the following physiological signals (pulse rate, heart rate variability, respiration rate and galvanic skin response). The subjective measurements were assessed using NASA-TLX and SAM tests after each task as it is shown in Figure 3.

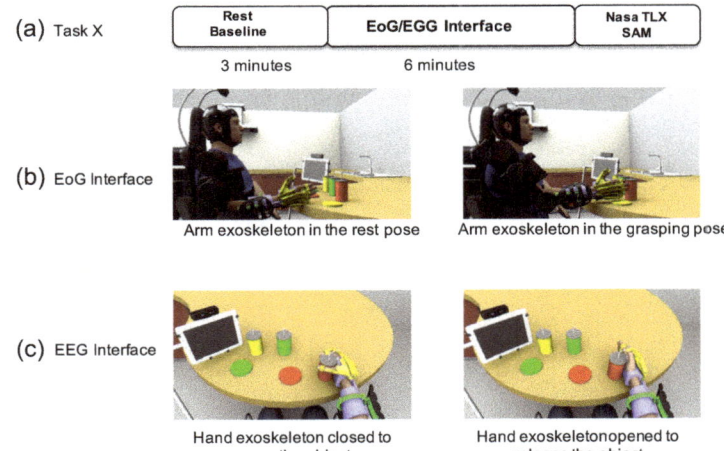

Figure 3. Experimental phase: (**a**) Each subject has to perform two tasks: one of them triggered by EoG interface and the other triggered by EEG interface (each task lasts 6 min). After completing each task, questionnaires were submitted to the user. After completing the questionnaires and before starting with a task, the subjects remain in a relaxed state for 3 min to obtain baseline measurements; (**b**) When the EoG trigger is detected, the exoskeleton moves from rest position to target object position computed by means of the RGB-D camera. Once the object is reached and the EoG trigger is detected, the exoskeleton moves to rest position. (**c**) EEG signal is used to command the closing of the hand exoskeleton. Once the hand is closed, EEG trigger is required to open the hand exoskeleton.

To compare the differences in the EEG and EoG interfaces, different analyses were carried out: correlation analysis to study the evolution of each signal with the time; and a statistical analysis (Mann–Whitney U test) to find differences between both interfaces. All these results are reported in the following subsections.

3.1. Interfaces and Performance

As it was explained before, none of the study participants had any prior experience in the use of these kind of interfaces. In the experiment, each participant was asked to perform two different activities using two interfaces: EEG and EoG. Both interfaces were used as a trigger to initiate the movements of the upper arm exoskeleton. Specifically, the activation time was defined as average time to detect a sensorimotor rhythm event-related desynchronization (SMR-ERD) for EEG interface and as average time to detect horizontal eye movements for EoG interface.

In particular, the EoG interface was used to initiate the exoskeleton movement from rest position to target object position computed by means of the RGB-D camera. Once the object is reached and the EoG trigger is detected, the exoskeleton moves to rest position. The mean success rate of EoG interface was 99.85% showing the reliability of the developed biosignal-processing algorithms to detect horizontal eye movements. Additionally, the mean activation time was 1.03 s.

On the other hand, the EEG interface was used to initiate the opening and closing movements of the hand exoskeleton. Once the hand is closed, EEG trigger is required to open the hand exoskeleton. The mean success rate of EEG interface was 63.75%. The mean activation time was 2.2 s.

Finally, the Mann–Whitney U test was used to compare the two interfaces, which showed a very significant difference ($p < 0.001$) for both performance and activation time. In Table 1, the descriptive statistics for both interfaces and results of the Mann–Whitney U test is presented.

Table 1. Descriptive statistics and results of Mann-Whitney U test between interfaces.

	Performance		Activation Time	
	EEG	EoG	EEG	EoG
Min.	21.43	96.77	1.55	0.85
1st Qu.	51.01	100.00	1.92	0.94
Median	65.71	100.00	2.10	1.02
Mean	63.75	99.85	2.20	1.03
3rd Qu.	79.09	100.00	2.46	1.11
Max.	93.75	100.00	3.20	1.25
Skewness	−0.58	−4.07	0.61	0.32
Kurtosis	−0.74	15.27	−0.44	−0.71
Mann-Whitney test p-value	<0.001		<0.001	

3.2. Physiological Measurements

Once the physiological signals were acquired, four features were extracted: pulse rate, respiration rate, heart rate variability and skin conductance level. Due to the high intra- and intersubject variability exhibited by psychophysiological responses, all these features were normalized by subtracting the actual value by the baseline value and then dividing the result by the baseline [35].

The Mann–Whitney U test was used to compare the physiological responses between using the two interfaces. In Figure 4, a statistically significant difference ($p < 0.05$) between both interfaces can be shown for both HRV and SCL signals. Pulse rate showed a trend to be higher in EEG tasks related to EoG tasks but the differences were not statistically significant. On the other hand, the respiration rate was very similar from both tasks.

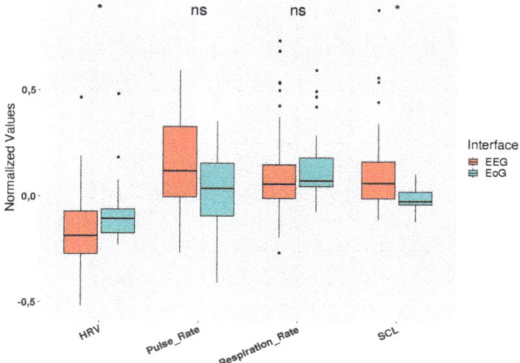

Figure 4. Changes in physiological signals between interfaces. HRV and SCL show a significant difference (* $p < 0.05$) between the two interfaces. Pulse rate shows a trend to be higher in EEG tasks related to EoG tasks.

In addition, an analysis of the changes over the time for each of the physiological features was performed. For this purpose, both tasks were divided into six periods of one minute in order to evaluate the different signals throughout the complete tasks. In Figure 5, this temporal analysis for both interfaces is presented, observing the mean physiological responses of all subjects during the tasks. Results of this analysis showed a similar behavior in each feature for both interfaces, though the trend in some cases is more pronounced in one of the interfaces. Specifically, these differences are more notable in HRV and SCL signals, where in the first case further decrease is observed for EEG task while in SCL a further decrease is observed for EoG.

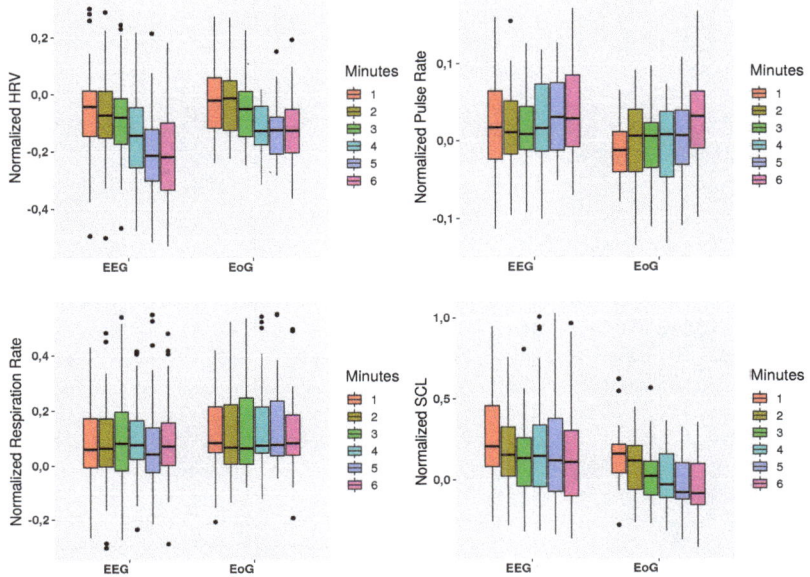

Figure 5. Temporal evolution of each physiological signal (HRV, SCL, respiration and pulse rate). They are shown for each minute (1, 2, 3, 4, 5, and 6 min) and interface (EEG vs. EoG).

Furthermore, a regression and statistical analysis were carried out to study the correlation between the changes in the different features of the physiological signals along the time of the task. In Table 2 results for Pearson correlation coefficient was computed, showing correlations in the decrease of the HRV along the time for both interfaces, as well as a decrease of the SCL for EoG interface. Moreover, the Wilcoxon Signed Rank test was carried out to compare the first and the last minutes for each feature, obtaining statistically significant differences for HRV and SCL for EEG interface and differences for HRV, pulse rate and SCL for EoG interface. These results are shown in the last column of Table 2.

Table 2. Temporal statistical results of the physiological signals: Pearson correlation between each signal and time is shown; as well as Wilcoxon Signed Rank test comparing the first and the last minute of each task.

		Pearson Correlation (signal vs. time)			Wilcoxon Signed Rank Test (minute 1 vs. minute 6)
		rho	R^2	p-Value	p-Value
EEG	HRV	−0.344	0.118	<0.001	<0.001
	Pulse Rate	0.134	0.018	0.030	0.064
	Resp. Rate	0.011	0.0001	0.865	0.544
	SCL	−0.086	0.007	0.234	<0.001
EoG	HRV	−0.339	0.115	0.001	0.011
	Pulse Rate	0.156	0.024	0.087	0.007
	Resp. Rate	0.016	0.0001	0.868	0.920
	SCL	−0.306	0.094	0.001	0.001

3.3. Subjective Ratings

To obtain the subjective perspective of the participants to compare and complete the information obtained with the physiological signals, two different well established questionnaires were completed immediately after each task by each operator: The NASA-TLX [36] and SAM [37] test.

The NASA-TLX is one of the most widely used to assess the subjective workload of the user through the use of six subscales: mental demand, physical demand, own performance, temporal demand, effort, and frustration. First, any possible paired-comparison of the subscales was conducted after each task for each subject. On the other hand, SAM test is an effective measure for self-report emotion recognition. Emotions are rated on a nine-point scale by the two dimensions valence and arousal. Each dimension is represented by nine graphic figures.

In Table 3 and Figure 6 the data reported by both questionnaires are shown. Additionally, results of a statistical test (Mann-Whitney U test) is also reported in order to compare both interfaces and the subjective perception for the participants. It can be observe that in almost all subjective parameters can be appreciate significant differences between the use of EEG and EoG. Only physical demand and temporal demand from NASA-TLX, and valence from SAM, do not show differences between interfaces; nevertheless, and showing Figure 6, in valence can be observed a slight trend to be higher in the use of EoG. In the same way, temporal demand indicates a slight trend to be higher in the use of EEG. It should be noted that the biggest difference can be observed in the perception of mental demand, much higher in the use of EEG over using EoG

Table 3. Report of questionnaires (mean ± STD) and statistical results of Mann-Whitney U test: all but three parameters (physical demand, temporal demand and valence) show significant differences between both interfaces.

Parameter	EEG		EoG		Mann-Whitney U Test
	Ratings	Scales	Ratings	Scales	p-Value
Mental Demand	13.23 ± 4.06	3.82 ± 2.86	4.05 ± 1.03	3.00 ± 1.15	<0.0001
Physical Demand	4.95 ± 3.56	6.55 ± 5.32	0.64 ± 0.89	3.36 ± 1.26	0.54
Temporal Demand	10.68 ± 2.99	8.82 ± 3.40	2.55 ± 1.35	3.10 ± 1.34	0.19
Performance	8.68 ± 4.10	2.36 ± 3.24	2.10 ± 0.86	0.45 ± 0.80	<0.001
Effort	12.00 ± 3.54	7.18 ± 4.55	2.91 ± 1.05	3.73 ± 1.08	0.007
Frustration	10.45 ± 5.34	2.73 ± 2.27	2.77 ± 1.70	1.36 ± 0.79	<0.001
Workload	58.38 ± 16.52		33.82 ± 14.78		<0.001
Valence	5.95 ± 1.56		6.82 ± 1.40		0.14
Arousal	3.95 ± 1.56		1.73 ± 1.01		<0.001

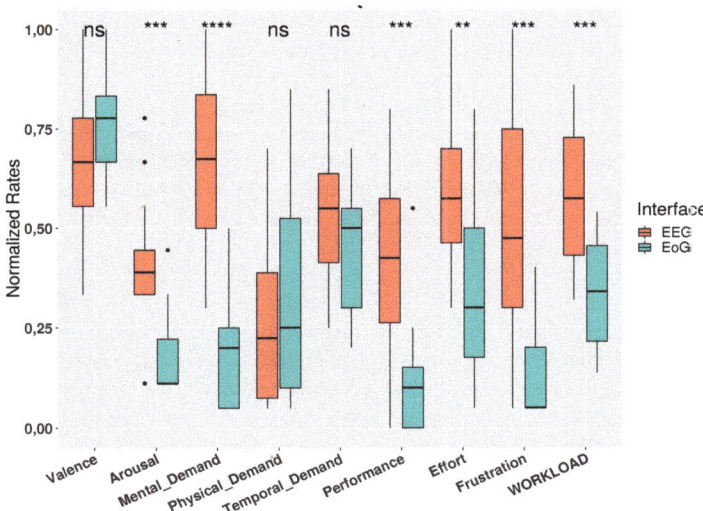

Figure 6. Normalized values of SAM and NASA-TLX tests for both interfaces (** $p<0.01$; *** $p<0.001$;**** $p<0.0001$)

4. Discussion

BNCI systems are mainly applied to two scenarios: brain/neural control of assistive devices, such as wearable robots and prostheses, and use of BNCI systems for rehabilitation [24,25]. Lately, the combination of both scenarios, the assistive and rehabilitation ones, was suggested to improve the user acceptability and adoption of BNCI systems [27]. In this context, the optimization of BNCI systems in terms of mental work load and user engagement accessible through the subject's physiological responses is a subject under investigation in this paper.

Specifically, the aim of our research is to study and analyze the subject's physiological responses to two different interfaces broadly used in Brain/neural-computer interfaces: EEG and EoG. The analysis of the use of them, and their responses in subject's physiological state, may lead to understand the best way to use these interfaces during an exhaustive task of hybrid BNCI. Specifically, in this work the subject's physiological responses are studied and analysed in the case of the use of a hybrid control interface to control an arm/hand exoskeleton for assisting people with disabilities on reaching and grasping objects.

Fatigue is a multidimensional entity, with behavioural, physiological and subjective dimensions, usually related to decreased alertness and increased drowsiness, and is usually accompanied by a reduction in motivation and impairment of task performance. Although mental fatigue is commonly observed following prolonged cognitive activity, its cognitive processes remain largely unknown.

In the literature different signals were demonstrated to be well-established indicators for cognitive workload and/or mental fatigue. Specifically, SCL is a generally well-established indicator of cognitive workload, which increases with mental demand of a task [38]. Furthermore, ECG is usually used as a physiological mark (computing HRV feature) relating its increase with mental fatigue [39,40]. Other studies [41], also suggest the existence of a coherent sequence of changes for EEG, EoG and heart rate variables during the transition from normal drive, high mental workload and eventually mental fatigue and drowsiness.

Our results are in line with these findings, where the temporal analysis shows differences in HRV and SCL from the first minute to the last minute of the tasks. In particular, it can be observe a slight more trend in the decrease of HRV for EoG interface, and a correlation between a decrease of SCL with time only in EoG tasks. Despite motor imagery task should be more intuitive for tasks, such as opening/closing a hand exoskeleton, than EoG, and these results suggest that the higher mental demand due to the motor imagery with respect to the pure physical activity of moving the eyes to one direction cause a higher mental fatigue in the use of EEG interface.

In addition, our results showed changes in HRV and SCL from the first to the last minutes of the task for each interface. There are statistically significant differences for HRV and SCL for EEG interface and differences for HRV, pulse rate and SCL for EoG interface. These findings could be the first step to adapt BNCI systems using changes in physiological reactions(e.g to dynamically adapt the bio-signal detection thresholds, etc.).

Regarding subjective rates, the differences in physiological signals between the use of both interfaces are consistent with the perceived workload resulting from NASA-TLX test.

These results suggest possible frustration and stress due to a long-time use of Hybrid BNCI. Since few studies [19–21] associate the user's psychological state with a performance decrease in brain-computer interface, understanding these physiological responses may lead us to develop adaptive techniques to detect and minimize this stress induced to the user by, for instance, changing between interfaces and using the most intuitive or the lesser mental demand one.

Furthermore, regression and statistical analyses were carried out to study the correlation between the changes in the different features of the physiological signals along the time of the task. In Table 2 results for Pearson correlation coefficient was computed, showing correlations in the decrease of the HRV along the time for both interfaces, as well as a decrease of the SCL for EoG interface. Moreover, Wilcoxon Signed Rank test was carried out to compare the first and the last minutes for each feature, obtaining statistically significant differences for HRV and SCL for EEG interface and differences for HRV, pulse rate and SCL for EoG interface. These results can be shown in the last column of Table 2.

5. Conclusions

Our main finding in this work is that the exhaustive use of BNCI interfaces produce subjects' quantitative changes in the physiological reactions in that subjects, and these changes are different for different interfaces: EEG and EoG. Specifically, our results suggest that HRV and SCL show significant differences between good and poor performance using both interfaces. Furthermore, the temporal analysis performed to the four physiological features processed, states a relationship between the amount of time exhaustively using the interfaces with the changes in the physiological response of the subjects. These analyses show a correlation between time and a decrease in HRV for both interfaces, which can indicate an increase in the level of stress of the subject's psychological state due to the exhaustiveness of the tasks. In addition, a correlation between time and a decrease in SCL is appreciated in the use of EoG, which can be explained with the lack of mental demand in the used of this interface.

In addition, our measured results are in accordance with the results of subject's workload perception and emotional responses assessed through NASA-TLX questionnaires and Self-Assessment Manikin(SAM) respectively.

This is the first step to adapt our Hybrid BNCI using changes in physiological reactions to customise the use of different interfaces during a long-time use of Hybrid BNCI, for instance changing between interfaces, with the aim of avoiding possible frustration and stress due to the high mental demand in EEG interfaces, which may lead to a decrease in the subject's performance.

Author Contributions: Conceptualization, S.C., S.R.S., L.Z. and N.G.-A.; Data curation, F.J.B. and J.A.D.; Formal analysis, J.M.C., E.T. and F.C.; Funding acquisition, N.G.-A.; Investigation, F.J.B., J.A.D., E.T., F.C., M.N., L.Z., N.V. and N.G.-A.; Methodology, S.C., S.R.S., L.Z., N.V. and N.G.-A.; Software, J.M.C., E.T. and M.N.; Supervision, N.G.-A.; Validation, J.M.C. and F.C.; Writing—original draft, F.J.B.; Writing—review & editing, S.R.S., N.V. and N.G.-A.

Funding: This research was funded by European Commission grant number 645322 and the Ministerio de Economía y Competitividad of Spain grant number DPI2015-70415-C2-R.

Conflicts of Interest: The authors declare no conflict of interest.

References

1. European Commision. People with disabilities have equal rights. In *The European Disability Strategy 2010–2020*; European Commision: Brussels, Belgium, 2010; ISBN:978-92-79-16836-9.
2. Müller-Putz, G.R.; Breitwieser, C.; Cincotti, F.; Leeb, R.; Schreuder, M.; Leotta, F.; Tavella, M.; Bianchi, L.; Kreilinger, A.; Ramsay, A.; et al. Tools for brain–computer interaction: A general concept for a hybrid BCI. *Front. Neuroinform.* **2011**, *5*, 30. [CrossRef] [PubMed]
3. Choi, I.; Rhiu, I.; Lee, Y.S.; Yun, M.W.; Nam, C.S. A Systematic Review of Hybrid Brain-Computer Interfaces: Taxonomy and Usability Perspectives. *PLoS ONE* **2017**, *12*, e0176674. [CrossRef] [PubMed]
4. Su, Y.; Qi, Y.; Luo, J.X.; Wu, B.; Yang, F.; Li, Y.; Zhuang, Y.T.; Zheng, X.X.; Chen, W.D. A hybrid brain-computer interface control strategy in a virtual environment. *J. Zhejiang Univ. Sci. C* **2011**, *12*, 351–361. [CrossRef]
5. Pan, J.; Xie, Q.; He, Y.; Wang, F.; Di H.; Laureys, S.; Yu, R.; Li, Y. Detecting awareness in patients with disorders of consciousness using a hybrid brain-computer interface. *J. Neural. Eng.* **2014**, *11*, 56007 [CrossRef] [PubMed]
6. Allison, B.Z.; Brunner, C.; Kaiser, V.; Muller-Putz, G.R.; Neuper, C.; Pfurtscheller, G. Toward a hybrid brain computer interface based on imagined movement and visual attention. *J. Neural. Eng.* **2010**, *7*, 026007. [CrossRef] [PubMed]
7. Úbeda, A.; Iáñez, E.; Badesa, J.; Morales, R.; Azorín, J.M.; García, N. Control strategies of an assistive robot using a Brain-Machine Interface. In Proceedings of the 2012 IEEE/RSJ International Conference on Intelligent Robots and Systems, Vilamoura, Portugal, 7–12 October 2012; pp. 3553–3558.
8. Yu, T.; Xiao, J.; Wang, F.; Zhang, R.; Gu, Z.; Cichocki, A.; Li, Y. Enhanced motor imagery training using a hybrid BCI with feedback. *IEEE Trans. Biomed. Eng.* **2015**, *62*, 1706–1717. [CrossRef] [PubMed]
9. Brunner, C.; Allison, B.Z.; Krusienski, D.J.; Mullerputz, G.R.; Pfurtscheller, G.; Neuper, C. Improved signal processing approaches in an offline simulation of a hybrid brain-computer interface. *J. Neurosci. Methods* **2010**, *188*, 165–173. [CrossRef] [PubMed]
10. Li, X.; Samuel, O.W.; Zhang, X.; Wang, H.; Fang, P.; Li, G. A motion-classification strategy based on sEMG-EEG signal combination for upper-limb amputees. *J. Neuroeng. Rehabil.* **2017**, *14*, 2. [CrossRef] [PubMed]
11. Kawase, T.; Sakurada, T.; Koike, Y.; Kansaku, K. A hybrid BMI- based exoskeleton for paresis: EMG control for assisting arm movements. *J. Neural Eng.* **2017**, *14*, 016015 [CrossRef] [PubMed]
12. Scherer, R.; Mller-Putz, G.R.; Pfurtscheller, G. Self-initiation of eeg-based brain-computer communication using the heart rate response. *J. Neural. Eng.* **2007**, *4*, L23–L29. [CrossRef] [PubMed]
13. Pfurtscheller, G.; Allison, B.Z.; Brunner, C.; Bauernfeind, G.; Escalante, T.S.; Scherer, R.; Zander, T.O.; Mueller-Putz, G.; Neuper, C.; Birbaumer, N. The hybrid bci. *Front. Neurosci.* **2010**, *4*, 30. [CrossRef] [PubMed]
14. Witkowski, M.; Cortese, M.; Cempini, M.; Mellinger, J.; Vitiello, N.; Soekadar, S.R. Enhancing brain–machine interface (BMI) control of a hand exoskeleton using electrooculography (EoG). *J. Neuroeng. Rehabil.* **2014**, *11*, 165. [CrossRef] [PubMed]
15. Surjo R. Soekadar, Matthias Witkowski, Nicola Vitiello, Niels Birbaumer An EEG/EoG-based hybrid brain-neural computer interaction (BNCI) system to control an exoskeleton for the paralyzed hand. *Biomed. Tech.* **2015**, *60*, 199–205. [CrossRef]
16. Frisoli, A.; Procopio, C.; Chisari, C.; Creatini, I.; Bonfiglio, L.; Bergamasco, M.; Rossi, B.; Carboncini, M. Positive effects of robotic exoskeleton training of upper limb reaching movements after stroke. *J. NeuroEng. Rehabil.* **2012**, *9*, 36. [CrossRef] [PubMed]
17. Barsotti, M.; Leonardis, D.; Loconsole, C.; Solazzi, M.; Sotgiu, E.; Procopio, C.; Chisari, C.; Bergamasco, M.; Frisoli, A. A full upper limb robotic exoskeleton for reaching and grasping rehabilitation triggered by MI-BCI. In Proceedings of the 2015 IEEE International Conference on Rehabilitation Robotics (ICORR), Singapore, 11–14 August 2015; pp. 49–54.
18. Pedrocchi, A.; Ferrante, S.; Ambrosini, E.G.; Olla, M.; Casellato, C.; Schauer, T.; Klauer, C.; Pascual, J.; Vidaurre, C.; Gfohler, M.; et al. Mundus project: MUltimodal neuroprosthesis for daily upper limb support. *J. Neuroeng. Rehabil.* **2013**, *10*, 6. [CrossRef] [PubMed]

19. Kaufmann, T.; Vögele, C.; Sütterlin, S.; Lukito, S.; Kübler, A. Effects of resting heart rate variability on performance in the P300 brain-computer interface. *Int. J. Psychophysiol.* **2012**, *83*, 336–341. [CrossRef] [PubMed]
20. Myrden, A.; Chau,T. Effects of user mental state on EEG-BCI performance. *Front. Hum.Neurosci.* **2015**, *9*, 308. [CrossRef] [PubMed]
21. Myrden, A.; Chau, T. A Passive EEG-BCI for Single-Trial Detection of Changes in Mental State. *IEEE Trans. Neural Syst. Rehabil. Eng.* **2017**, *25*, 345–356. [CrossRef] [PubMed]
22. Mohammadpour, M.; Mozaffari, S. Classification of EEG-based attention for brain computer interface. In Proceedings of the 2017 3rd Iranian Conference on Intelligent Systems and Signal Processing (ICSPIS), Shahrood, Iran, 20–21 December 2017; pp. 34–37.
23. Li, Y.; Li, X.; Ratcliffe, M.; Liu, L.; Qi, Y.; Liu, Q. A real-time EEG-based BCI system for attention recognition in ubiquitous environment. In Proceedings of the 2011 International Workshop on Ubiquitous Affective Awareness and Intelligent Interaction (UAAII '11), Beijing, China, 18 September 2011; pp. 33–40.
24. Ushiba, J.; Soekadar, S.R. Brain-machine interfaces for rehabilitation of poststroke hemiplegia. *Prog. Brain Res.* **2016**, *228*, 163–183. [PubMed]
25. Soekadar, S.R.; Birbaumer, N.; Slutzky, M.W.; Cohen, L.G. Brain-Machine Interfaces in Neurorehabilitation of Stroke. *Neurobiol. Dis.* **2015**, *83*, 172–179; [CrossRef] [PubMed]
26. Soekadar, S.R.; Witkowski, M.; Gómez, C.; Opisso, E.; Medina, J.; Cortese, M.; Cempini, M.; Carrozza, M.C.; Cohen, L.G.; Birbaumer, N.; et al. Hybrid EEG/EoG-based brain/neural hand exoskeleton restores fully independent daily living activities after quadriplegia. *Sci. Robot.* **2016**, *1*, eaag3296. [CrossRef]
27. Soekadar, S.R.; Nann, M.; Crea, S.; Trigili, E.; Gómez, C.; Opisso, E.; Cohen, L.G.; Birbaumer, N.; Vitiello, N. Restoration of Finger and Arm Movements Using Hybrid Brain/Neural Assistive Technology in Everyday Life Environments. In *Brain-Computer Interface Research*; Guger, C., Mrachacz-Kersting, N., Allison, B., Eds.; SpringerBriefs in Electrical and Computer Engineering; Springer: Cham, Switzerland, 2019.
28. Crea, S.; Nann, M.; Trigili, E.; Cordella, F.; Baldoni, A.; Badesa, F.J.; Catalán, J.M.; Zollo, L.; Vitiello, N.; Aracil, N.G.; et al. Feasibility and safety of shared EEG/EOG and vision-guided autonomous whole-arm exoskeleton control to perform activities of daily living. *Scienfic Rep.* **2018**, *8*, 10823. [CrossRef] [PubMed]
29. Pfurtscheller, G.; da Silva, L.F.H. Event-related EEG/MEG synchronization and desynchronization: Basic principles. *Clin. Neurophysiol.* **1999**, *110*, 1842–1857. [CrossRef]
30. Toyama, S.; Takano, K.; Kansaku, K. A non-adhesive solid-gel electrode for a non-invasive brain-machine interface. *Front. Neurol.* **2012**, *3*, 114. [CrossRef] [PubMed]
31. McFarl, D.J. The advantages of the surface Laplacian in brain-computer interface research. *Int. J. Psychophysiol.* **2015**, *97*, 271–276. [CrossRef] [PubMed]
32. Crea, S.; Cempini, M.; Moisè, M.; Baldoni, A.; Trigili, E.; Marconi, D.; Cortese, M.; Giovacchini, F.; Posteraro, F.; Vitiello, N. A novel shoulder-elbow exoskeleton with series elastic actuators. In Proceedings of the 6th IEEE International Conference on Biomedical Robotics and Biomechatronics (BioRob), Singapore, 26–29 June 2016; pp. 1248–1253.
33. Trigili, E.; Crea, S.; Moisè, M.; Baldoni, A.; Cempini, M.; Ercolini, G.; Marconi, D.; Posteraro, F.; Carrozza, M.C.; Vitiello, N. Design and Experimental Characterization of a Shoulder-Elbow Exoskeleton with Compliant Joints for Post-Stroke Rehabilitation. *IEEE/ASME Trans. Mechatron.* **2019**, *24*, 1485–1496. [CrossRef]
34. Díez, J.A.; Blanco, A.; Catalán, J.M.; Badesa, F.J.; Lledó, L.D.; García-Aracil, N. Hand exoskeleton for rehabilitation therapies with integrated optical force sensor. *Adv. Mech. Eng.* **2018**, *10*, 2. [CrossRef]
35. Novak, D.; Mihelj, M.; Munih, M. A survey of methods for data fusion and system adaptation using autonomic nervous system responses in physiological computing. *Interact. Comput.* **2012**, *24*, 154–172. [CrossRef]
36. NASA. *Nasa Task Load Index (TLX) v. 1.0 Manual*; NASN: Washington, DC, USA, 1986.
37. Bradley, M.M.; Lang, P.J. Measuring emotion: The self-assessment manikin and the semantic differential. *J. Behav. Ther. Exp Psychiatry* **1994**, *25*, 49–59. [CrossRef]
38. Collet, C.; Averty, P.; Dittmar, A. Autonomic nervous system and subjective ratings of strain in air-traffic control. *Appl. Ergon.* **2009**, *40*, 23–32. [CrossRef] [PubMed]
39. Egelund, N. Spectral analysis of heart rate variability as an indicator of driver fatigue. *Ergonomics* **1982**, *25*, 663–672. [CrossRef] [PubMed]

40. Mascord, D.J.; Heath, R.A. Behavioral and physiological indices of fatigue in a visual tracking task. *J. Saf. Res.* **1992**, *23*, 19–25. [CrossRef]
41. Borghini, G.; Astolfi, L.; Vecchiato, G.; Mattia, D.; Babiloni, F. Measuring neurophysiological signals in aircraft pilots and car drivers for the assessment of mental workload, fatigue and drowsiness. *Neurosci. Biobehav. Rev.* **2014**, *44*, 58–75. [CrossRef] [PubMed]

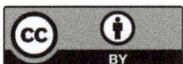 © 2019 by the authors. Licensee MDPI, Basel, Switzerland. This article is an open access article distributed under the terms and conditions of the Creative Commons Attribution (CC BY) license (http://creativecommons.org/licenses/by/4.0/).

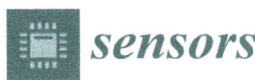

Article

Pseudo-Online BMI Based on EEG to Detect the Appearance of Sudden Obstacles during Walking

María Elvira, Eduardo Iáñez *, Vicente Quiles, Mario Ortiz and José M. Azorín

Brain-Machine Interface Systems Lab, Miguel Hernández University of Elche, Avda. de la Universidad S/N, Ed. Innova, Elche, 03202 Alicante, Spain; maria.elvira01@goumh.umh.es (M.E.); vquiles@umh.es (V.Q.); mortiz@umh.es (M.O.); jm.azorin@umh.es (J.M.A.)
* Correspondence: eianez@umh.es; Tel.: +34-965-22-2271

Received: 30 September 2019; Accepted: 5 December 2019; Published: 10 December 2019

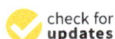

Abstract: The aim of this paper is to describe new methods for detecting the appearance of unexpected obstacles during normal gait from EEG signals, improving the accuracy and reducing the false positive rate obtained in previous studies. This way, an exoskeleton for rehabilitation or assistance of people with motor limitations commanded by a Brain-Machine Interface (BMI) could be stopped in case that an obstacle suddenly appears during walking. The EEG data of nine healthy subjects were collected during their normal gait while an obstacle appearance was simulated by the projection of a laser line in a random pattern. Different approaches were considered for selecting the parameters of the BMI: subsets of electrodes, time windows and classifier probabilities, which were based on a linear discriminant analysis (LDA). The pseudo-online results of the BMI for detecting the appearance of obstacles, with an average percentage of 63.9% of accuracy and 2.6 false positives per minute, showed a significant improvement over previous studies.

Keywords: Brain-Machine Interface (BMI); EEG; obstacle; gait

---

1. Introduction

The rate of individuals affected by a motor disability is increasing due to the aging of the population and the growing number of chronic diseases, standing at 15% of the world population, according to the World Health Organization (WHO). It has been shown that rehabilitation treatment in the first six months after a stroke or a spinal cord injury is the most effective way to recover lost mobility, due to the plasticity of the nervous system during this time [1]. At this stage, however, traditional rehabilitation presents great difficulties for many patients because of their inability to perform the relevant movements or because of the excessive physical effort that therapy requires. For this reason, the use of exoskeletons during rehabilitation therapies presents great benefits. In addition, the use of Brain-Machine Interfaces (BMIs) allow a greater involvement of the patient during his/her rehabilitation and, consequently, a better recovery [2].

BMIs based on electroencelographic (EEG) signals record the brain activity in a non-invasive way and translate brain signals into commands for controlling external devices [3]. BMIs have been applied in rehabilitation for controlling upper-limb prosthetics [4,5]. In relation to the development of BMIs for commanding lower-limb exoskeletons, EEG signals have been analyzed in order to detect mental states related to walking [6].

On one hand, patients can use an exoskeleton in the chronic phase to be assisted in movement [7,8]. This allows them to increase their independence and mobility. On the other hand, the acute phase of rehabilitation is when a better improvement of the functional capabilities of a patient can be acquired. Therefore, the combination of an exoskeleton and BMI could also be useful during therapy, due to the cognitive involvement of the users, with a more intuitive, clear and dynamic control.

EEG signals can be used for obtaining relevant information about patient intentions or specific motor mental processes. In this regard, several works analyze the detection of starting or stopping gait from EEG signals based on voluntary intention of the user [9–11]. Continuous gait motor imagination has also been used as a paradigm to control the gait of an exoskeleton [12].

Moreover, there are other mental processes of interest which could be useful in controlling an exoskeleton, such as the detection of speed changes or direction changes [13]. All the former research has been used to create commands to control an exoskeleton. However, the reliability of the BMIs must increase before extended real-time applications, and especially the false positive rates must be reduced.

Another important aspect when commanding an exoskeleton is to keep high safety conditions. In the case that an unexpected obstacle appears, it is necessary to stop the device as soon as possible. Exoskeletons used to have an emergency button for this purpose, but it requires an active action by the subject. This action is not instinctive and it could be affected by the medical condition of the subject and by response time. An alternative option could be the integration of an automatic image processing system to detect obstacles and generate the stop command [14]. However, this option requires additional hardware and it is more computationally extensive. Moreover, it requires not only the detection of the obstacles, but also the interpretation of whether or not it is an obstacle that really requires a stop. For example, Bi et al. use a vision system to detect obstacles during driving situations [15]. In this work, the visual system is also combined with obstacle detection through EEG signals.

The use of cerebral information is based on the detection of different potential patterns when an obstacle appears and the person voluntarily decides to react by stopping or not. This analysis could allow a transparent detection by the subject, performing the detection faster than the user's physical reaction. Some studies have already analyzed brain signals through error-related potentials (ERPs), studying visually in the frequency domain the response to an obstacle between aggressive and gentle drivers when using a driving simulator [16]. If the detection is performed soon enough after perceiving the obstacle, an emergency stop can be performed, improving safety. This includes not only the visualization of the obstacle, but also the decision to react to it. Therefore, it is the person who will determine the type of reaction to the obstacle, avoiding the need of interpretation by the system that visual paradigms require.

The detection of the intention of a subject to stop after the appearance of an unexpected obstacle has been analyzed in previous works [17,18]. In these previous studies, brain signals were analyzed when an unexpected external disturbance appeared while walking on a treadmill. The disturbance was simulated by a laser line and the user had to suddenly stop their gait in response to the obstacle. It was found that when averaging several events, a potential appeared in the electrodes of the fronto-central area before the real stop of the user, allowing anticipation of the actual stop. However, those events must be detected in a single trial in order to generate commands in real time. The offline analysis of the features of the potential through common spatial patterns (CSP), slope or polynomial fit allowed the classification by linear discriminant analysis (LDA) with a maximum accuracy of 80%. As a last step, a pseudo-online analysis with a sliding window of a half second to detect the events was performed. Even if the initial results were promising, the false positive rate still remained very high (6.7) and accuracy dropped to 30% [17]. A low false positive rate would allow someone to send a stop command to an exoskeleton in the case of an emergency event, making possible its implementation in real time in a reliable, useful and safe way [19].

The goal of this work is to significantly improve the results of previous work. Inertial measurement units (IMUs) are used to measure the real moment of a stop in order to compare it with the detection of a stop intention by the system. Moreover, new methods have been explored for personalizing the electrode selection and to determine the data window with more relevant information for the model creation. New features allow a better differentiation between the potential after and before the event. Results are tested by a pseudo-online analysis which provides a more similar approach to future real-time implementation with an exoskeleton. The paper shows the pseudo-online results obtained by nine healthy subjects.

2. Materials and Methods

The following section describes the software and hardware that have been used in the experiments, as well as the experimental procedure. This includes: the methods used for pre-processing the EEG signals, extraction of features, and their classification. Furthermore, the methods used for an accurate monitoring of the movement of the person through inertial measurement units (IMUs) are also detailed. Finally, the strategy used to get the pseudo-online results is also defined.

2.1. Experimental Set-Up

Two commercial amplifiers (g.USPamp from the g.Tec company, Graz, Austria) have been used for registering the EEG signals. Each amplifier registers 16 input channels, so a total of 32 electrodes are registered at a sampling frequency rate of 1200 Hz. The amplifiers include a notch hardware filter at 50 Hz. Both devices have been synchronized using the g.INTERsync module. The electrode distribution follows the International System 10/10 [20], and they are distributed over the scalp following this order: Fz, FC5, FC1, FCz, FC2, FC6, C3, Cz, C4, CP5, CP1, CP2, CP6, P3, Pz, P4, PO7, PO3, PO4, PO8, FC3, FC4, C5, C1, C2, C6, CP3, CPZ, CP4, P1, P2 and POz. The reference has been positioned on the right ear lobe, and AFz is used as ground.

Furthermore, the Tech MCS V3 equipment from Technaid (Arganda del Rey, Spain) has been used for monitoring the movement of the subject. The IMUs are used to detect the moment when the subject actually stops. This allows researchers to mark the time of the windows of analysis for the moments prior to the obstacle appearance and when the subject reacts to the stimulus and stops. The Tech MCS V3 device uses 7 IMUs, registering up to 19 parameters such us acceleration or gyros at a frequency sample of 30 Hz. They are distributed in the body as follows: one IMU is placed on the lumbar area, and three IMUs are placed on each leg on the right/left thigh, right/left shin and right/left foot.

Both EEG signals and motion information are registered and synchronized using a Matlab API. Matlab has also been used for data processing and analysis.

Additionally, a treadmill Pro-form Performance 750 has been used to keep a constant and controlled velocity during the trials. A laser line projected onto the front of the treadmill, with a wavelength of 635 nm (red color) and an output power of 3 mW, has been used to simulate the appearance of sudden obstacles. The laser line is activated by a trigger out of the g.USBamp device, which also allows labelling of the EEG events. Figure 1 shows the experimental set-up.

2.2. Experimental Procedure

The experimental procedure is as follows:

1. First, the full procedure is explained to the subjects and all the equipment is set up. Subjects see how the obstacle appearance works through laser activation. Before the experiment starts, subjects get used to stopping when they see the laser line appear. As the treadmill is moving slowly, it is safe to stop for a second and a half and to resume their gait without falling from the platform. Nevertheless, a safety belt is set on the subject to stop the treadmill automatically if the subject moves a certain distance backwards. In addition, a researcher in charge of the experiment is placed behind the treadmill during the experiment to avoid any possible unsafe situation.
2. Then, subjects perform 10 trials to complete a full session. For each trial, the next steps are followed:

    - First, the subject stands on the treadmill without any movement, while the software is connected to the g.Tec equipment and the IMUs are calibrated.
    - Next, the subject starts walking on the treadmill at a constant velocity of 2 km/h and 0 degrees of inclination. Once the person is walking safely and in a stable manner, the data acquisition starts.

- Each trial lasts 2 min. During this time, the laser line is projected randomly during one second. The interval between two successive stimuli varies between six and nine seconds. Therefore, the total number of lasers that appear on each trial is between 12 and 14. The subject is instructed to suddenly stop when the laser is visualized and then resume gait after a couple of seconds as previously explained.

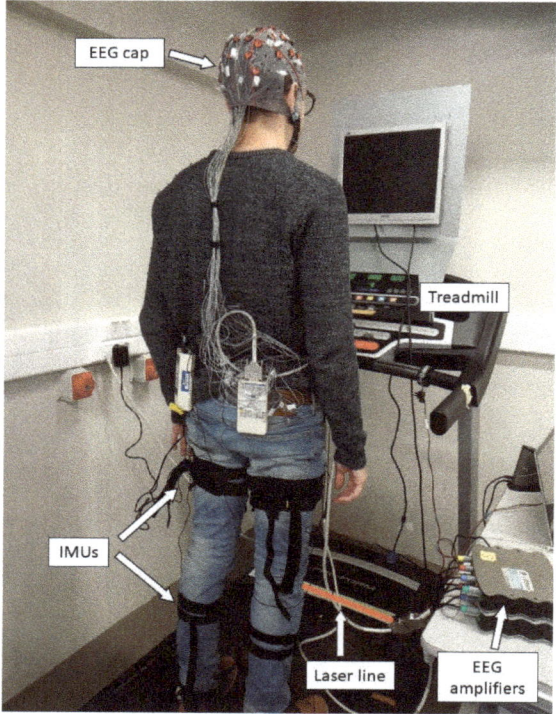

Figure 1. Experimental set-up. The subject stands on the treadmill wearing the inertial measurement units (IMUs) for registering movement and the electroencelographic (EEG) cap for registering EEG signals. The subject keeps a normal gait of 2 km/h for 2 min, while a laser line is projected randomly onto the front of the treadmill.

2.3. Stop Detection Method Through IMUs

As mentioned before, 7 IMUs have been distributed on the body. The module of the acceleration of the axes X, Y and Z (3 of the 19 outputs of the IMUs) is calculated. After that, the continuous wavelet transform (CWT) [21], with a scale range of 1:64 is applied. Then, a parameter is calculated as the sum of the CWT coefficients in the range 3:30 (where the frequency components of interest are).

In order to make a decision, an initial threshold is needed. This is determined as the mean of the parameter of the first trial of each subject. Each trial is analyzed with a sliding window of 20 samples (0.67 s) shifted at a 3 samples pace (0.1 s). If the parameter computed for each window is less than half of the threshold, then it is considered that there is a significant decrease in the signal, and a stop is computed. As the windows analysis overlaps, a detection is only considered if there is a significant decrease in the current epoch and not in the previous one. Finally, the threshold is updated for each window, averaging it with the signal value of the previous window.

2.4. Offline Model Creation

This subsection shows the different steps and alternatives considered to create the model for classification of the EEG signals: preprocessing, electrode selection, time window selection and classification. Figure 2 (left) shows a general diagram of the procedure applied.

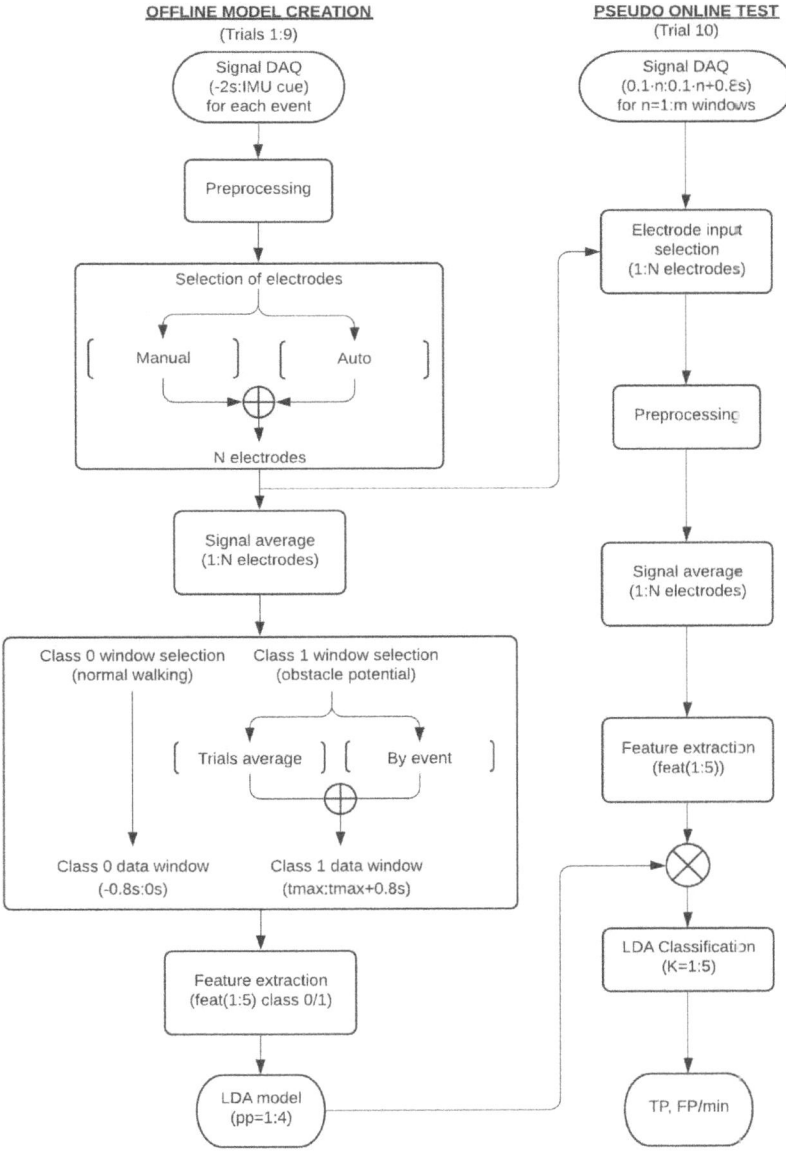

Figure 2. General scheme of the EEG signal acquisition applied to each window. Left shows the procedure for the offline model creation. Right shows the pseudo-online test procedure.

First, in order to create a suitable model that allows the detection of obstacles, it is important to determine a proper window of analysis. This window must cover the time from when the subject is walking normally to when an actual stop is detected by the IMUs. Then, the electrode information corresponding to this period of time is preprocessed and subsequently the selection of a significant group of electrodes is averaged for them. Two different classes are considered for the model creation, depending on the performed action: normal walking (class 0) and response to the obstacle (class 1). For each event of an obstacle appearance, features are extracted from the data of both classes for model creation. The trials considered for model creation correspond to the first 9 trials of a session (Figure 2, left), leaving the 10th trial for testing the model in a pseudo-online scenario (Figure 2, right). In the case of the pseudo-online analysis, the preprocessing is only applied to the personalized selection of electrodes of each subject obtained during the model creation.

2.4.1. Preprocessing

In the case of the model creation, for each event, the period of analysis starts 800 ms before the laser activation and ends before the IMU's detection of the stop. To increase the noise-to-signal ratio some preprocessing must be applied to the signals.

Based on a previous work where motion artifacts were analyzed during walking conditions, it was concluded that the noise is mainly focused on peripheral areas corresponding to the scalp locations more sensitive to conductivity changes [22]. Moreover, in this previous work, periphery electrodes were discarded after analyzing all the electrodes and verifying that they were more affected by artifacts due to cap features, e.g., poor contact with the scalp when walking [17].

This is why, from the initial 32 electrodes, those located on the periphery of the head, and therefore more possibly affected by movement artifacts, have been discarded: FC5, FC6, CP5, CP6, PO3, PO4, PO7, PO8, C5 and C6.

Then, to the remaining 22 electrodes, a band-pass filter from 0.4 to 3 Hz has been applied as the studied potentials are in a low-frequency range. Finally, in order to remove possible artifacts, those signals with standard deviation greater than 40 µV have been removed. This is an important aspect to assure that the model creation uses only suitable EEG information.

2.4.2. Selection of Electrodes

There are four main lobes in the brain: frontal, temporal, parietal and occipital [23]. The EEG pattern to be looked for corresponds with the response to an unexpected visual stimulus, which is also associated with the intention of stopping. Therefore, the brain areas of interest for analysis are the motor, sensory and occipital area, which are located respectively in the frontal, parietal and occipital lobes. After removing the peripheral electrodes indicated in Section 2.4.1, the remaining 22 electrodes are part of the aforementioned areas. This way, the electrodes registered are: Fz, FC1, FCz, FC2, C3, Cz, C4, CP1, CP2, P3, Pz, P4, FC3, FC4, C1, C2, CP3, CPz, CP4, P1, P2, POz.

However, not all the electrodes are used for the classifier and a subset of the electrodes is selected based on the magnitude of the variation of the potential after a laser activation (Figure 2, left). This selection has been carried out in two different ways: manual and automatic.

The manual selection method consists of visual observation of the signals after the laser appearance for each electrode. The selected electrodes are the ones that from inspection show a higher distinctive potential. This procedure takes usually less than five minutes. Figure 3 represents an example of the inspected signals for one of the subjects and shows the comparison between the averaged signal (black line) obtained by choosing the 22 electrodes (a), and the one obtained by manual selection (b). It can be seen that after manual selection, the averaged signal is more homogeneous and there is a more significant change after the laser line appearance (red line) and before the real physical stop of the subject determined by the IMUs (cyan line).

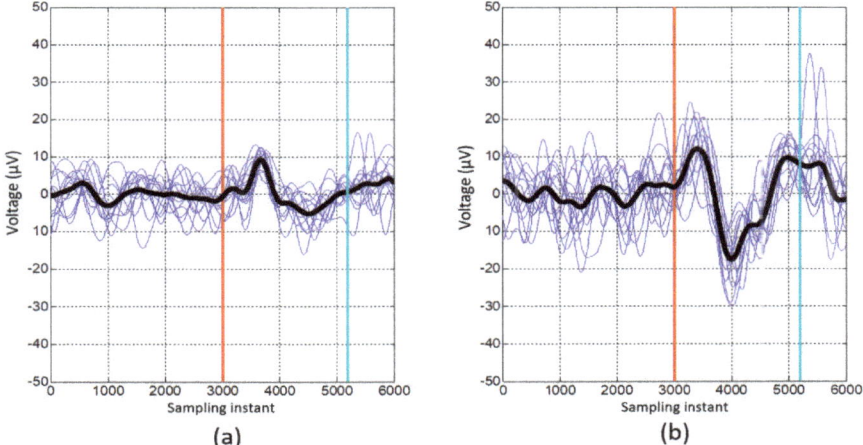

Figure 3. Comparison between the signal obtained by choosing all the electrodes of the mentioned areas (a), and the one obtained including only the signal of the electrodes chosen individually (b). On the X axis, the sampling time for a frequency of 1200 Hz appears. On the Y axis the value of the voltage in µV is represented. The laser appears at the sampling instant 3000 (at 2.5 s) and is represented by the red vertical line, picking up the signal for the 2.5 s before the laser and the 2.5 s after. In addition, the vertical line in cyan blue represents the moment in which the real stop of the person occurs (averaging all the stops made in the session represented and detected by IMUs).

The automatic selection of the electrodes tries to reproduce the previous criteria. The objective is to eliminate those electrodes that contribute less to the expected potential. The procedure of this automatic selection method can be defined as follows:

1. The procedure starts with the preprocessed signals from −2 s to the IMU's cue for each event and the 22 electrodes (N = 22).
2. N different combinations of electrodes, discarding one electrode for each combination, are analyzed.
3. For each combination, all N−1 electrodes are averaged for each individual event each time the laser line appears (similarly to the black line in Figure 3).
4. As the pattern expected is a first positive deflection followed by a negative deflection, the method locates the first maximum voltage ($max_{láser}$) after the laser appearance, and locates the minimum voltage ($min_{láser}$) in the first second after this maximum. In addition, the maximum voltage (max_{walk}) and the minimum voltage (min_{walk}) of the signal during the two seconds of normal walking before the laser appearance are also calculated. These values are assessed for each of the laser activations. After that, the relation between the amplitude of the signal after and before the laser is obtained as:

$$dif = \frac{max_{láser} - min_{láser}}{max_{walk} - min_{walk}} * 100 \qquad (1)$$

5. Then, a single value for each of the combinations of the electrodes is calculated as:

$$dif_{total} = \text{average}(dif) - \text{standard deviation }(dif) \qquad (2)$$

6. Next, the maximum dif_{total} value (corresponding to a certain configuration of electrodes) is analyzed. If this maximum value is higher than the maximum value from the previous iteration (for the first iteration it would be compared to the original 22 combination), the electrode not participating in the combination is discarded and N = N−1.

7. This process (steps 2 to 6) is repeated for successive N–1 combinations of electrodes, i.e., while the first iteration tests combinations of 21 electrodes, the second tests for combinations of 20 electrodes, third of 19 and so on.
8. Iteration stops when the maximum dif_{total} of the iteration has a lower value than the one from the previous iteration.
9. In order to be sure that the removed electrodes are not relevant, a second revision is performed.
10. This second revision is done through trying a subset of electrodes, discarding one by one the discarded electrodes. Steps 2–5 are repeated keeping the electrode only if its dif_{total} is higher than the one obtained by Step 8, or definitively discarding it if its lower.

2.4.3. Personalized Selection of Time Windows

According to the conclusions obtained in [17], it is known that after a visual stimulus is followed by a reaction, a positive deflection in the EEG signal 700 ms before the reaction of the person, followed by a negative deflection 400 ms before that reaction, can be observed. However, high variability between people's reaction times should be considered. Therefore, in order to select a suitable time window for modeling the EEG potentials and for improving the results, the time window is selected for each subject individually (Figure 2, left). That is when the greatest variation of the amplitude of the EEG signal is observed. This will improve model creation.

Figure 4a,b show, as an example, the temporary lag between two subjects, S8 and S6. The electrodes selected in the previous step are averaged and each laser activation is shown together with the average. While in the first case the maximum of the average signal is produced 150 ms after the laser, for the second case the maximum is located at 685 ms. Considering this situation, two possible solutions are proposed for selecting the beginning of the class 1 window.

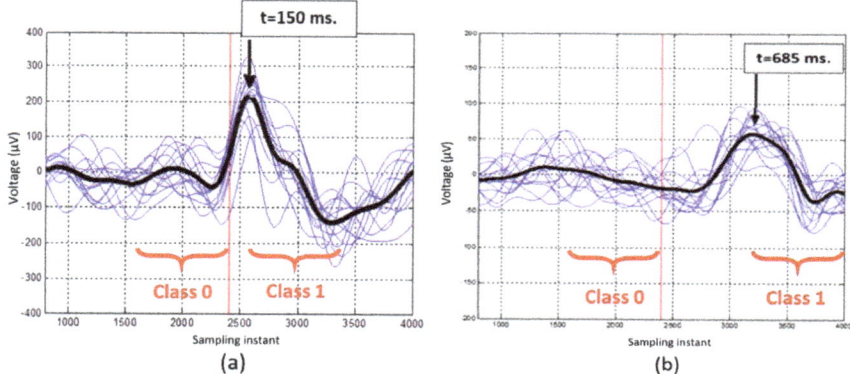

Figure 4. Temporary lag between the positive deflection in subjects S8 (**a**) and S6 (**b**). The sampling time (f = 1200 Hz) is represented on the X axis. The amplitude of the signal obtained by adding the potential in the electrodes chosen for each subject individually, in µV, is represented on the Y axis. The blue lines represent this sum signal in different laser activations of the same session and in black are the average of all of them. The vertical red line represents the appearance of the laser.

The first alternative consists of calculating on average the moment in which the greatest variation in the amplitude of the EEG signal occurs. This is calculated by obtaining the average of all events (as shown in Figure 4), and detecting the moment of the maximum of this average signal.

The second alternative tries to create a personalized model, locating the maximum of the signal in each event in the range of 2 s after the laser appearance.

Therefore, the time window that represents the class 1 (laser) for obtaining the model will be chosen starting in the time when the maximum is detected and will have a length of 800 ms. In contrast, the time window of class 0 (non-laser) will be chosen equally for all subjects lasting also 800 ms just before the laser appearance. This way, the area of greatest difference between class 1 (laser) and class 0 (non-laser) can be captured.

2.4.4. Feature Extraction

After the selection of the subset of electrodes and the 800 ms time windows for class 0 and 1, feature extraction is performed (Figure 2, left). In all cases, the features have been obtained from the average of the signal of the electrodes chosen for each subject, which is called $f1$.

From this signal $f1$, a vector with 5 features has been extracted:

1. Area included under the curve of the absolute value of $f1$ derivative:

$$feat(1) = \int abs(f1') \quad (3)$$

2. Variance of $f1$ derivative:

$$feat(2) = var(f1') \quad (4)$$

3. Amplitude of $f1$ derivative:

$$feat(3) = max(f1') - min(f1') \quad (5)$$

4. Amplitude of the accumulative sum of the absolute value of $f1$ along a window:

$$feat(4) = max(sum(f1)) - min(sum(f1)) \quad (6)$$

5. Maximum cross correlation between $g1$ and $f1$ in each case ($g1$ is the mean of all the $f1$ obtained in each particular laser appearance):

$$feat(5) = max(f1 \star g1)_i \quad (7)$$

The features vector is obtained for all window classes 0 and 1, and is properly labelled.

2.4.5. Classifier

For the distinction between the 2 classes, a linear discriminant analysis (LDA) has been chosen as the classifier, which transforms a set of α-dimensional data into a δ-dimensional subspace (with $\delta < \alpha$), maximizing the distance between the means of each class and, simultaneously, minimizing their dispersions [24,25] (Figure 2e).

The discrimination function is as follows:

$$h_\beta(x) = \begin{cases} (\beta^T \cdot x + \beta_o) \geq 0 \rightarrow 1 \\ (\beta^T \cdot x + \beta_o) < 0 \rightarrow 2 \end{cases} \quad (8)$$

$$\beta = \sum^{-1}(\mu_1 - \mu_2) \quad (9)$$

$$\beta_o = -\beta^T \cdot \left(\frac{\mu_1 + \mu_2}{2}\right) + ln\left(\frac{\pi_1}{\pi_2}\right) \quad (10)$$

where β is the vector of classification parameters, β_o is the bias term, $\sum$ is the clustered covariance matrix, μ_1 and μ_2 are the average vectors of class 1 and class 2, and π_1 and π_2 are their prior probabilities [26]. As these probabilities are not known a priori, they are also analyzed in the results section for a prior probability (π) assigned to class 0 of $\pi = 1:4$ versus $\pi = 1$ to class 1.

2.5. Pseudo-Online Analysis

In order to achieve a more realistic evaluation of the BMI, a pseudo-online classification is performed using the last trial of each session.

For this purpose, a sliding window from EEG signals of 0.8 s has been analyzed, shifting each one by 0.1 s. Each window was analyzed following the procedure in Figure 2 (right) and is classified as to whether it belongs to an event of walking (class 1) or response to the obstacle (class 0).

The process is applied only to the electrodes selected during the model creation. Since the band-pass filter can distort the sides of short time windows, the length of the window is extended to the previous seconds of each moving window. Then, after applying the band-pass filter, only the last 0.8 s are kept for the next steps. Then, the data of the selected electrodes are averaged and their features are extracted. Finally, the LDA model is applied to obtain the classification of each moving window as class 0 or 1.

Due to the overlapping of windows (0.7 s), there is redundant information that can cause the detection of several successive windows as class 1, when for instance only one has been produced [27]. Therefore, a K value that represents the number of positive detections (class 1), must be taken into account to assure a correct one. This parameter has been tested for values of K from 1 to 5. For example, if an isolated detection is performed with K = 2, it will not be considered, as it would require at least 2 consecutive detections to its computation. A correct selection of K helps to reduce the number of false positives.

In addition, the real-time algorithm for detecting the stop through the Tech MCS equipment described in Section 2.3 has been included in the pseudo-online test. Due to the structure of the test, when the person restarts the gait after a stop, a noise is generated on the EEG signal. This distortion affects the BMI system, as it could be detected as a false positive. However, as the obstacle detection must be only considered when the subject is walking, the predicted class is automatically set to 0 during the windows associated with the 1.5 s after the IMU's detection of a stop. This period of time is not considered for the total count of seconds, in order to not affect the FP/min rate.

2.6. Subjects

Nine healthy subjects, with ages between 21 and 54 years, without any neurological disorders and with normal vision have participated in the experiments. The experiments were approved by the Ethics Committee of the Miguel Hernández University of Elche (Spain). All subjects were informed and signed informed consent according to the Helsinki declaration.

3. Results

This section starts describing the results of the stop detection through the IMUs. This is a critical result, as the feedback of the IMUs provides the tool used for the definition of a real physical stop. Section 3.2 shows the subset of electrodes obtained by manual selection as explained in Section 2.4.2. From Section 3.3 onwards, the results cover the different analysis considered for the detection of the stop intention through EEG. Results are obtained from the pseudo-online analysis of the last trial of each session. The parameters computed include the true positive rate (TP) and the false positive rate (FP/min). The different subsections correspond to some of the alternative paths shown in Figure 2. The first default analysis (Section 3.2) uses a manual selection of electrodes, the average of trials for the window selection of class 1, a prior probability of 4 and K values from 1 to 5. From those default results, successive analyses study alternative paths such as changing the prior probability of the classifier, selecting the class 1 windows by event or using an automatic selection of the electrodes. Finally, the time of detection by the algorithm is compared to the time when the stop is computed by the IMUs, in order to assure that the detection is assessed before the real stop happens.

3.1. Results of the Stop Detection through the IMUs

Table 1 shows, for each subject, the percentage of stops correctly detected through IMUs (TP: true positive) and the percentage of stops not detected (FN: false negative). Both values have been calculated on average for all the sessions of each subject. The number of false positives is also included, considering FP as the cases where a stop is detected but there is not a real one. Furthermore, the average time for each subject to detect the stop from the laser activation is shown.

Table 1. Results of stop detection through IMUs.

Subject	TP (%)	FP (%)	Average Time (s)
S1	92.3 ± 5.1	0.0	1.9
S2	82.7 ± 9.9	0.0	2.0
S3	99.2 ± 2.4	0.0	1.8
S4	88.1 ± 11.5	0.0	2.1
S5	95.9 ± 8.1	0.6	1.9
S6	82.3 ± 10.0	0.1	2.1
S7	96.9 ± 4.0	0.0	1.6
S8	96.2 ± 9.8	0.0	1.6
S9	99.2 ± 2.6	0.0	1.9
Mean ± σ	92.5 ± 7.0	0.1 ± 0.2	1.9 ± 0.2

From the results, it can be asserted that the algorithm properly detects the stops, with a TP percentage of 92.5% ± 7.0% and only 0.1 ± 0.2 FP. There are only false detections for 2 of the subjects (S5 and S6) while the rest of them have 0 false detections.

Regarding the reaction time for each subject, the values are in the range of 1.6 to 2.1, which could be considered a high variability range. In this sense it must be considered that all the subjects do not stop in the same way. Some of them stop their gait immediately after seeing the laser, while others go one step further before stopping. This could explain this variability, in addition to the different reaction times of each person.

It is important to remark that the objective of the research is to detect the intention of the subject to stop when an obstacle appears. Therefore, the time showed in Table 1 must be lower than the needed time by the developed algorithm to detect a stop intention.

3.2. Manual Electrode Selection

Table 2 shows the list of electrodes selected for each subject with the manual method. Furthermore, the maximum of the average signal is included in the third column, in milliseconds, determined by the addition of the selected electrodes in all laser appearances.

Table 2. Manual electrode selection and maximum location for each subject. Electrodes coincidental with automatic electrode selection in bold text.

Subject	Manual Electrode Selection	Maximum Location (ms)
S1	Fz, FC1, **FCz, FC2**, Cz, P1	465.8
S2	Fz, FC1, FCz, **FC2**, CP1, Pz, P4	329.3
S3	Fz, FCz, Cz, POz	414.2
S4	Fz, FC1, FCz, FC2, C3, Cz, CP1, CP2, P3, Pz, FC3, C1, C2, CP3, CPz	719.2
S5	Fz, FC1, FCz, **FC2**, Cz, C4, **P1**	547.5
S6	C4, CP2, Pz, **P4**	665.8
S7	Fz, **FC1**, FCz, Cz, CP2	501.7
S8	Fz, **FC1**, FCz, FC2, C3, Cz, C4, CP1, CP2, P3	132.5
S9	Fz, FC1, FCz, FC2, **P1**, P2	523.3

From the results some conclusions can be obtained. First, in 8 out of 9 subjects there is an activation of the electrode FCz, which reflects that an error-related potential is being generated when the obstacle appears [28]. Also, electrodes Cz and Fz, located in the same area (fronto-central area) appear in most of the subjects. Additionally, there is an activation of the motor area, with the inclusion of electrodes such as FCz, FC2, C1, C2, C3 and C4 due to the intention of a stop. Finally, the occipital electrodes such as P1, P2, P3, P4, POz and Pz are also activated due to the visualized obstacle. Both behaviors could be expected since we have a visual stimulus (laser), to which the subject reacts, sending an order to stop.

3.3. Results of the Pseudo-Online Analysis with Initial Configuration

Table 3 shows the results obtained in the pseudo-online analysis of the tenth trial. The default configuration considered is based on the manual electrode selection and the time windows selection for class 1 after the maximum time showed in Table 2. The prior probability assigned to class 0 (non-laser) is 4 versus 1 for class 1 (laser).

Table 3. Results for the pseudo-online analysis with different values of K. Best values according the criteria (bold).

	K = 2		K = 3		K = 4		K = 5	
Subject	TP	FP/min	TP	FP/min	TP	FP/min	TP	FP/min
S1	69.2	8.8	61.5	4.4	69.2	2.9	38.5	1.5
S2	46.2	4.9	**30.8**	**1.4**	7.7	0.0	0.0	0.0
S3	69.2	7.5	**69.2**	**3.7**	61.5	1.5	46.2	0.7
S4	46.2	4.3	**30.8**	**2.9**	7.7	2.2	7.7	0.0
S5	76.9	7.7	61.5	5.1	**66.7**	**0.0**	30.8	0.0
S6	76.9	6.7	76.9	4.4	**61.5**	**2.2**	38.5	0.7
S7	38.5	8.1	**23.1**	**3.7**	7.7	3.0	0.0	3.0
S8	92.9	7.2	**92.9**	**3.6**	85.7	2.9	35.7	0.7
S9	**91.7**	**3.8**	83.3	1.5	66.7	0.8	25.0	0.0

A detection is considered successful when it happens in the interval between the appearance of the obstacle and the average reaction of the subject. The pseudo-online analysis is calculated for K values between 1 and 5. Results for K = 1 are not detailed in the tables since the FP/min are too excessive to be considered as acceptable.

The criteria which has been followed for considering the best result is to keep a FP/min rate lower than 4 with the highest TP value. Following this rule, Table 3 shows in bold text the best result for each case and subject. Results show a mean TP value of 59.5% ± 25.9% and an average value FP/min rate of 2.7 ± 1.3 The K values depend on the subjects with values from 2 to 4.

3.4. Results Varying the Prior Probability of the Classifier

Table 4 shows the comparison between the TP and FP/min rates for different values of prior probability π = 2:4 assigned to class 0 (non-laser) versus π = 1 to class 1. To condense the information, only the results of the optimum K value are shown for each subject.

Table 4. Results obtained in the pseudo-online analysis for different values of prior probability for class 1 (laser).

Subject	Probability π = 2			Probability π = 3			Probability π = 4		
	K	TP	FP/min	K	TP	FP/min	K	TP	FP/min
S1	5.0	53.8	3.7	5.0	46.2	2.2	4.0	69.2	2.9
S2	4.0	38.5	3.5	4.0	23.1	0.7	3.0	30.8	1.4
S3	5.0	69.2	3.0	4.0	69.2	3.0	3.0	69.2	3.7
S4	5.0	53.8	2.2	3.0	46.2	2.9	3.0	30.8	2.9
S5	4.0	66.7	2.6	4.0	66.7	0.0	4.0	66.7	0.0
S6	5.0	76.9	2.2	4.0	76.9	3.0	4.0	61.5	2.2
S7	4.0	15.4	3.7	5.0	15.4	3.0	3.0	23.1	3.7
S8	5.0	57.1	1.4	4.0	92.9	3.6	3.0	92.9	3.6
S9	4.0	83.3	2.3	3.0	91.7	2.3	2.0	91.7	3.8
Mean ± σ	4.6	57.2 ± 19.5	2.7 ± 0.8	**4.0**	**58.7 ± 26.3**	**2.3 ± 1.1**	3.0	58.7 ± 24.2	2.7 ± 1.2

Results for equal prior probabilities (1 vs. 1) for both classes have not been included because of the high FP/min obtained by all the subjects.

According to these results, prior probability of 3 for the class 0 offers the best relation between TP and FP/min rate, so the next analysis will use this probability to calculate the results.

3.5. Results when Modifications are Made to the Best Case

The results in this subsection take into account two alternatives regarding time window selection and automatic electrode selection.

3.5.1. Results for Time Windows of Class 1 Obtained from a Particularized Maximum by Event

Table 5 shows the results obtained for capturing the time windows for class 1 locating the maximum of the signal for each time window, according to the explanation given in Section 2.4.3. Results are generally worse with this alternative, except for the subject S1, who obtains a significant improvement. For the rest of the subjects TP has a value of 46.6% ± 27.8% and FP/min of 2.7 ± 0.8. This reflects a decrease of nearly a 15% in the obstacle detection, while the FP/min rate only decreases by 0.1. Therefore, it is not worthwhile to particularize the class 1 window by event.

Table 5. Results for capturing the time windows with the particularized maximum.

Subject	K = 2		K = 3		K = 4		K = 5	
	TP	FP/min	TP	FP/min	TP	FP/min	TP	FP/min
S1	76.9	11.7	69.2	6.6	61.5	3.7	38.5	2.9
S2	38.5	12.0	23.1	2.8	7.7	0.7	7.7	0.0
S3	69.2	11.9	61.5	6.7	53.8	4.5	53.8	3.0
S4	38.5	4.3	23.1	2.9	7.7	2.2	0.0	1.4
S5	83.3	8.5	66.7	6.8	25.0	0.9	16.7	0.0
S6	92.3	14.8	76.9	7.4	61.5	3.0	23.1	0.7
S7	8.3	4.4	8.3	2.2	8.3	1.5	0.0	0.7
S8	92.9	7.2	85.7	5.8	85.7	5.1	71.4	2.9
S9	91.7	3.8	91.7	3.0	58.3	1.5	33.3	0.0

3.5.2. Results Obtained with the Automatic Selection Electrodes

Table 6 shows the list of the electrodes obtained with the automatic selection as it was explained in Section 2.4.2, as well as the time instance from which the time window for class 1 is captured for creating the model, according to the mean obtained from all the laser appearances.

Table 6. List of electrodes obtained with the automatic method for each subject. Electrodes coincidental with manual electrode selection in bold text.

Subject	Automatic Electrode Selection	Sample Instant (ms)
S1	Fz, FC2, Cz, CP1, Pz, P4, P1	482.5
S2	Fz, FC2, P3, Pz, P4	337.5
S3	Fz, FC1, FCz, Cz	386.7
S4	Fz, C4, P4, CP4, P1, P2, POz	710.0
S5	Fz, FC2, P1	698.0
S6	FC1, Cz, P4	789.2
S7	Fz, FC1, C4	148.3
S8	Fz, FC1, CP4, P1	151.7
S9	Fz, P3, P4, P1, POz	485.0

If this selection is compared with the one obtained manually, it can be seen that with the automatic method, in 8 out of 9 cases the selection includes a lower or equal number of electrodes. Additionally, as it happens with the manual selection, the electrodes that appear more frequently are again the ones related to the error-related potential: FCz, Fz (which appear in all the subjects), Cz, FC1 and FC2. The electrodes located in the occipital zone (P1, P2, P3, P4, POz and Pz), where visual information is generated, also seem to contribute to the generation of a distinctive potential in most of the cases. Electrodes located in the motor area (C1, C2, C3 and C4), appear only in subject S7, so the potential generated for the stop intention is weaker, contributing less to the detection of the potential in the automatic selection method.

Table 7 shows the results obtained with the pseudo-online analysis. Only the results for the best value of K are shown. The right side of the table shows the best results obtained with the manual selection method for comparison.

Table 7. Comparison between the results obtained with the automatic electrode selection and with the manual selection.

Subject	Optimal Case with Automatic Selection			Optimal Case with Manual Selection		
	K	TP	FP/min	K	TP	FP/min
S1	4	61.5	2.9	5	46.2	2.2
S2	3	46.2	3.5	4	23.1	0.7
S3	4	69.2	3.0	4	69.2	3.0
S4	5	30.8	2.9	3	46.2	2.9
S5	4	83.3	2.6	4	66.7	0.0
S6	4	61.5	0.0	4	76.9	3.0
S7	-	-	-	5	15.4	3.0
S8	4	100.0	3.6	4	92.9	3.6
S9	3	69.2	3.8	3	91.7	2.3

It is difficult to consider which electrode selection performs better. Two out of the ten subjects, S1 and S8, improve with the automatic selection. However, in the case of S4 and S9, the results get considerably worse. Subject S3 obtains exactly the same rates, while in the rest of the cases it is not clear as to whether the results improve or worsen, because a TP rate increase is correlated to a higher FP/min and vice versa.

As a criterion for its application in real time, the electrode selection could be first done using the automatic selection, as it is an unsupervised, faster method. After the model and selection is created, a new trial could be done to see if the TP is higher than 60% and the FP/min is lower than 3.0. If they are, the automatic selection is used, and if not a supervised manual selection is done and tested in pseudo-online analysis to see if the results could be improved.

3.6. Analysis of Instant Time Detection Versus Obstacle Appearance and Physical Stop Detection

In this subsection the instance after the laser appearance, when the BMI detects the intention to make a stop through EEG signals, is analyzed. This instant is compared with the instant when the IMUs detect the stop. With the difference between these two moments it can be stated whether the stop intention is detected before the real stop of the person. For instance, this could be helpful in the command of an exoskeleton, allowing the subject to stop it faster than the reaction time.

Table 8 shows those results taking into account the optimal value of K obtained for each subject with a prior probability $\pi = 3$ for the class 0 and with the manual selection of electrodes. The time interval between the detection of a stop through the IMUs and the classification of class 1 through the BMI (2nd column) are shown. Table 8 also shows the interval between the obstacle appearance and the obstacle detection through the BMI (3rd column). Both intervals are calculated averaging all the time differences obtained with the different laser appearances. In all the cases, the detection of the potential has been produced before the real detection by the person. This means that the BMI has been able to predict the detection of the subject.

Table 8. Analysis of the instant time detection (in seconds): IMUs vs. Brain-Machine Interface (BMI), which indicates prediction time before physical stop of the user; and BMI vs. laser appearance, which indicates how much time the BMI needs in order to detect the stop after the obstacle appears suddenly through the laser.

Subject	IMUs Detection–BMI Detection	BMI Detection–Obstacle Appearance
S1	0.8 ± 0.1	1.2 ± 0.1
S2	1.9 ± 0.1	1.1 ± 0.2
S3	0.7 ± 0.2	1.2 ± 0.1
S4	0.7 ± 0.4	1.5 ± 0.4
S5	0.9 ± 0.5	1.3 ± 0.5
S6	0.8 ± 0.2	1.2 ± 0.2
S7	0.4 ± 0.0	0.9 ± 0.0
S8	0.8 ± 0.2	0.9 ± 0.1
S9	0.7 ± 0.2	1.2 ± 0.1
Mean ± σ	0.9 ± 0.2	1.2 ± 0.2

The average anticipation is 0.9 ± 0.2 s, which could be considered enough anticipation to send a command to an exoskeleton and stop it in the case of an obstacle appearance.

Regarding the time interval between the laser appearance and the detection through the EEG signals, an averaged value of 1.2 ± 0.2 s is obtained. In this case, however, a great variability between subjects is shown. In fact, it must be appreciated that there is a relation between the instant when the maximum of the EEG signal was observed in each subject and the mean value when the intention to stop is being detected through the pseudo-online analysis. For instance, in S4 the peak of the signal appears 720 ms after the laser appearance (the highest value) and has the highest time interval (1.5 s).

4. Conclusions

This paper has evaluated new methodologies for detecting the appearance of unexpected obstacles while walking using EEG signals. Since the final goal is to propose a method that can be used in real-time tests, the chosen alternative cannot involve excessive time for training the BMI system and obtaining the model. That is why it has been decided to personalize some of the algorithm decisions, due to the improvement of the results, and generalize others to reduce the time needed to create the model. The results have been tested in a pseudo-online scenario which is a more realistic analysis and is suitable for its future application in combination with an exoskeleton in real time.

Regarding the selection of the electrodes it is not possible to conclude which method, manual or automatic, achieves better results. Therefore, the criterion consists of applying the automatic faster selection in an initial stage, and depending on the results obtained, applying a second manual selection for trying to improve the results. The selection of the class 1 data for the model creation performs better when it is based on the maximum of the average signal of all events per subject instead of personalizing it by event. The results of applying different prior probabilities for the LDA classifier indicates that $\pi = 3$ is the most beneficial one in general terms for the class 0. Finally, the K value for consecutive detections should be personalized during the model creation between values of 2 and 5 for each subject, since the results vary widely depending on the subject.

Following all these considerations, the best results obtained for each subject according to all the tested variations are shown in right part of Table 9. The second column (M/A) indicates if a manual or automatic solution for electrode selection has been followed. This allows us to compare the results with previous work [17], showed in the left part of Table 9, where a polynomial feature extraction was performed. A significant improvement in the percentage of true positives can be observed, from 30.0% to 63.9%, and also a clear reduction in the FP/min (from 6.7 to 2.6). In addition, it is possible to affirm that the BMI system is capable of detecting the intention to stop of the person in a time prior to the actual stop, sufficient enough to be able to send an order to the exoskeleton in a reasonable time.

Table 9. Comparison between the bests results obtained with previous research.

Previous Research [17]				Current Research				
Subject	K	TP (%)	FP/min	Subject	M/A	K	TP (%)	FP/min
S1	4	28.6	8.0	S1	A	4	61.5	2.9
S2	4	42.9	2.1	S2	A	3	46.2	3.5
S3	2	42.9	8.5	S3	A	4	69.2	3.0
S4	2	7.1	2.7	S4	M	3	46.2	2.9
S5	2	28.6	11.9	S5	A	4	83.3	2.6
				S6	A	4	61.5	0.0
				S7	M	5	15.4	3.0
Mean ± σ		30.0 ± 14.6	6.7 ± 4.2	S8	A	4	100.0	3.6
				S9	M	3	91.7	2.3
				Mean ± σ			63.9 ± 26.2	2.6 ± 1.1

Future works will focus on performing real-time experiments by applying the procedure in order to move to the final stage by testing this architecture with an exoskeleton. It will also be analyzed if a lower number of trials to create the model allows us to obtain similar or better results in order to decrease the needed training time. However, there is still work to do in order to increase success percentage and to reduce as much as possible the FP/min. This is the most critical parameter for its implementation with an exoskeleton.

Author Contributions: Conceptualization, M.E., E.I., M.O. and J.M.A.; methodology, M.E., V.Q. and E.I.; software, M.E., V.Q. and E.I.; validation, M.E., V.Q. and M.O.; formal analysis, M.E.; investigation, M.E. and V.Q.; resources, M.E., J.M.A.; Data curation, M.E., E.I. and M.O.; writing–original draft preparation, M.E. and E.I.; writing–review and editing, E.I., M.O. and J.M.A.; visualization, M.E.; supervision, E.I. and J.M.A.; project administration, J.M.A.; funding acquisition, J.M.A.

Funding: This research has been carried out in the framework of the project Walk—Controlling lower-limb exoskeletons by means of brain-machine interfaces to assist people with walking disabilities (RTI2018-096677-B-I00), funded by the Spanish Ministry of Science, Innovation and Universities, the Spanish State Agency of Research, and the European Union through the European Regional Development Fund.

Acknowledgments: We want to thank all the subjects that took part in the experiments.

Conflicts of Interest: The authors declare no conflict of interest. The funders had no role in the design of the study; in the collection, analyses, or interpretation of data; in the writing of the manuscript, or in the decision to publish the results.

References

1. Murie-Fernández, M.; Irimia, P.; Martínez-Vila, E.; Meyer, M.J.; Teasell, R. Neuro-rehabilitation after stroke. *Neurología (Engl. Ed.)* **2010**, *25*, 189–196. [CrossRef]
2. Wada, K.; Ono, Y.; Kurata, M.; Ito, M.I.; Minakuchi, M.T.; Kono, M.; Tominaga, T. Development of a Brain-machine Interface for Stroke Rehabilitation Using Event-related Desynchronization and Proprioceptive Feedback. *Adv. Biomed. Eng.* **2019**, *8*, 53–59. [CrossRef]
3. Wolpaw, J.R.; Birbaumer, N.; McFarland, D.J.; Pfurtscheller, G.; Vaughan, T.M. Brain–computer interfaces for communication and control. *Clin. Neurophysiol.* **2002**, *113*, 767–791. [CrossRef]
4. Fitzsimmons, N.A.; Lebedev, M.A.; Peikon, I.D.; Nicolelis, M.A. Extracting kinematic parameters for monkey bipedal walking from cortical neuronal ensemble activity. *Front. Integr. Neurosci.* **2009**, *3*, 1–19. [CrossRef] [PubMed]
5. Dollar, A.M.; Herr, H. Lower extremity exoskeletons and active orthoses: Challenges and state-of-the-art. *IEEE Trans. Robot.* **2008**, *24*, 144–158. [CrossRef]
6. Presacco, A.; Goodman, R.; Forrester, L.; Contreras-Vidal, J.L. Neural decoding of treadmill walking from noninvasive electroencephalographic signals. *J. Neurophysiol.* **2011**, *106*, 1875–1887. [CrossRef] [PubMed]
7. Yeung, L.F.; Ockenfeld, C.; Pang, M.K.; Wai, H.W.; Soo, O.Y.; Li, S.W.; Tong, K.Y. Randomized controlled trial of robot-assisted gait training with dorsiflexion assistance on chronic stroke patients wearing ankle-foot-orthosis. *J. Neuroeng. Rehabil.* **2018**, *15*, 51. [CrossRef]
8. Rajasekaran, V.; López-Larraz, E.; Trincado-Alonso, F.; Aranda, J.; Montesano, L.; Del-Ama, A.J.; Pons, J.L. Volition-adaptive control for gait training using wearable exoskeleton: Preliminary tests with incomplete spinal cord injury individuals. *J. Neuroeng. Rehabil.* **2018**, *15*, 4. [CrossRef]

9. Sburlea, A.I.; Montesano, L.; Minguez, J. Continuous detection of the self-initiated walking pre-movement state from EEG correlates without session-to-session recalibration. *J. Neural Eng.* **2015**, *12*, 036007. [CrossRef]
10. Jiang, N.; Gizzi, L.; Mrachacz-Kersting, N.; Dremstrup, K.; Farina, D. A brain–computer interface for single-trial detection of gait initiation from movement related cortical potentials. *Clin. Neurophysiol.* **2015**, *126*, 154–159. [CrossRef]
11. Lisi, G.; Morimoto, J. EEG single-trial detection of gait speed changes during treadmill walk. *PLoS ONE* **2015**, *10*, e0125479. [CrossRef] [PubMed]
12. Del Castillo, M.D.; Serrano, J.I.; Lerma, S.; Martínez, I.; Rocón, E. Neurophysiologic Assessment of Motor Imagery Training by Using Virtual Reality for Pediatric Population with Cerebral Palsy. *Revista Iberoamericana de Automática e Informática Industrial* **2018**, *15*, 174–179. [CrossRef]
13. Hortal, E.; Úbeda, A.; Iáñez, E.; Azorín, J.M.; Fernández, E. EEG-based Detection of Starting and Stopping During Gait Cycle. *Int. J. Neural Syst.* **2016**, *26*, 1650029. [CrossRef] [PubMed]
14. He, Y.; Eguren, D.; Azorín, J.M.; Grossman, R.G.; Luu, T.P.; Contreras-Vidal, J.L. Brain–machine interfaces for controlling lower-limb powered robotic systems. *J. Neural Eng.* **2018**, *15*, 021004. [CrossRef] [PubMed]
15. Bi, L.; Wang, H.; Teng, T.; Guan, C. A Novel Method of Emergency Situation Detection for a Brain-Controlled Vehicle by Combining EEG Signals with Surrounding Information. *IEEE Trans. Neural Syst. Rehabil. Eng.* **2018**, *26*, 1926–1934. [CrossRef]
16. Lin, C.T.; Liang, S.F.; Chao, W.H.; Ko, L.W.; Chao, C.F.; Chen, Y.C.; Huang, T.Y. Driving style classification by analyzing EEG responses to unexpected obstacle dodging tasks. In Proceedings of the 2006 IEEE International Conference on Systems, Man and Cybernetics, Taipei, Taiwan, 8–11 October 2006; Volume 5, pp. 4916–4919.
17. Salazar-Varas, R.; Costa, Á.; Iáñez, E.; Úbeda, A.; Hortal, E.; Azorín, J.M. Analyzing EEG signals to detect unexpected obstacles during walking. *J. Neuroeng. Rehabil.* **2015**, *12*, 101. [CrossRef]
18. Salazar-Varas, R.; Costa, A.; Úbeda, A.; Iáñez, E.; Azorín, J.M. Changes in brain activity due to the sudden apparition of an obstacle during gait. In Proceedings of the 2015 7th International IEEE/EMBS Conference on Neural Engineering (NER), Montpellier, France, 22–24 April 2015; pp. 110–113.
19. Lebedev, M.A.; Nicolelis, M.A. Brain–machine interfaces: Past, present and future. *TRENDS Neurosci.* **2006**, *29*, 536–546. [CrossRef]
20. Chatrian, G.E.; Lettich, E.; Nelson, P.L. Ten Percent Electrode System for Topographic Studies of Spontaneous and Evoked EEG Activities. *Am. J. EEG Technol.* **1985**, *25*, 83–92. [CrossRef]
21. Mallat, S.; Hwang, W.L. Singularity detection and processing with wavelets. *IEEE Trans. Inf. Theory* **1992**, *38*, 617–643. [CrossRef]
22. Costa, Á.; Salazar-Varas, R.; Úbeda, A.; Azorín, J.M. Characterization of Artifacts Produced by Gel Displacement on Non-invasive Brain-Machine Interfaces during Ambulation. *Front. Neurosci.* **2016**, *10*, 60. [CrossRef]
23. Cramer, S.C.; Lastra, L.; Lacourse, M.G.; Cohen, M.J. Brain motor system function after chronic, complete spinal cord injury. *Brain* **2005**, *128*, 2941–2950. [CrossRef]
24. Webb, A.R. *Statistical Pattern Recognition*; John Wiley & Sons: Hoboken, NJ, USA, 2003.
25. Fukunaga, K. *Introduction to Statistical Pattern Recognition*; Academic Press: Cambridge, MA, USA, 2013; pp. 131–153.
26. Bellingegni, A.D.; Gruppioni, E.; Colazzo, G.; Davalli, A.; Sacchetti, R.; Guglielmelli, E.; Zollo, L. NLR, MLP, SVM, and LDA: A comparative analysis on EMG data from people with trans-radial amputation. *J. Neuroeng. Rehabil.* **2017**, *14*, 82. [CrossRef]
27. Iáñez, E.; Costa, A.; Úbeda, A.; Rodríguez-Ugarte, M.; Azorín, J.M. A new upgrading model for detecting the reaction to obstacle appearance during walking using EEG. In Proceedings of the XXXVII Jornadas de Automática, Madrid, Spain, 7–9 September 2016; pp. 184–189.
28. Costa, A.; Hortal, E.; Úbeda, A.; Iáñez, E.; Azorín, J.M. Reducing the False Positives Rate in a BCI System to Detect Error-Related EEG Potentials. In *Replace, Repair, Restore, Relieve—Bridging Clinical and Engineering Solutions in Neurorehabilitation, Proceedings of the 2nd International Conference on NeuroRehabilitation (ICNR 2014), Aalborg, Denmark, 24–26 June 2014*; Spring: Cham, Switzerland, 2004; Volume 7, pp. 321–327. [CrossRef]

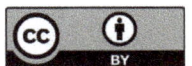

© 2019 by the authors. Licensee MDPI, Basel, Switzerland. This article is an open access article distributed under the terms and conditions of the Creative Commons Attribution (CC BY) license (http://creativecommons.org/licenses/by/4.0/).

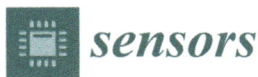

Article

AMiCUS—A Head Motion-Based Interface for Control of an Assistive Robot

Nina Rudigkeit *,† and Marion Gebhard

Group of Sensors and Actuators, Department of Electrical Engineering and Applied Physics, Westphalian University of Applied Sciences, 45877 Gelsenkirchen, Germany; marion.gebhard@w-hs.de
* Correspondence: publications.rudigkeit@gmail.com
† Current address: Xsens Technologies B.V., P.O. Box 559, 7500 AN Enschede, The Netherlands.

Received: 23 May 2019; Accepted: 18 June 2019; Published: 25 June 2019

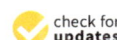

Abstract: Within this work we present AMiCUS, a Human-Robot Interface that enables tetraplegics to control a multi-degree of freedom robot arm in real-time using solely head motion, empowering them to perform simple manipulation tasks independently. The article describes the hardware, software and signal processing of AMiCUS and presents the results of a volunteer study with 13 able-bodied subjects and 6 tetraplegics with severe head motion limitations. As part of the study, the subjects performed two different pick-and-place tasks. The usability was assessed with a questionnaire. The overall performance and the main control elements were evaluated with objective measures such as completion rate and interaction time. The results show that the mapping of head motion onto robot motion is intuitive and the given feedback is useful, enabling smooth, precise and efficient robot control and resulting in high user-acceptance. Furthermore, it could be demonstrated that the robot did not move unintendedly, giving a positive prognosis for safety requirements in the framework of a certification of a product prototype. On top of that, AMiCUS enabled every subject to control the robot arm, independent of prior experience and degree of head motion limitation, making the system available for a wide range of motion impaired users.

Keywords: assistive technology; human-machine interaction; motion sensors; robot control; tetraplegia; IMU; AHRS; head control; gesture recognition; real-time control

1. Introduction

Tetraplegia is defined as the partial or total loss of motor and/or sensory function of the arms, legs, trunk and pelvic organs due to damage of the cervical segments of the spinal cord [1]. Besides traumatic injuries also disorders like cerebral palsy, amyotrophic lateral sclerosis or multiple sclerosis can lead to this severe disability [2]. The worldwide incidence of tetraplegia is estimated to lie between 3.5 and 27.7 per million inhabitants per year. The percentage of tetraplegics of all cases of spinal cord injuries increased within the last decades [3].

Tetraplegic patients require extensive home care services and often retire from working life because they no longer meet the physical conditions. The development of assistive robots for the people concerned is of major importance to at least partly restore their autonomy, substantially improving their quality of life.

Different uni- or multimodal Human–Machine Interface (HMI) concepts for tetraplegics have already been tested. These interfaces consider the user's remaining capabilities to voluntarily produce input signals, such as movement of eyes [4], head [5] or tongue [6], speech [7], breath [8], brain activity [9] or voluntary muscle contraction of neck [10], facial [11] or ear muscles [12]. The choice of the most suitable input modality depends on the preferences and physical abilities of each user as well as on the underlying control scheme. However, the goal of the research presented here was developing a solely head motion-based interface for real-time control of a robotic arm.

Common sensing modalities for head motion are ultrasound modules [13], ordinary cameras [14], infrared cameras, chin joysticks [15] and motion sensors [16]. In recent years, state-of-the-art motion sensors, such as Attitude Heading Reference Systems (AHRS) based on Micro Electro-Mechanical Systems (MEMS) technology, have gained increasing interest because they enable accurate motion measurement while being small, low-cost, lightweight, energy-efficient and self-contained, making them ideal for use in HMIs. For this reason, a MEMS AHRS has been considered the preferred choice to measure head motion within this work.

The majority of existing motion sensor-based head-controlled interfaces are limited to 2D-applications, such as control of mouse cursors [16–20], wheelchairs [17,21] or other vehicles [5]. Few attention has been paid to more complex applications, such as robot arm control. However, Williams et al. [22] use head orientation to control the Tool Center Point (TCP) of a robot arm. Furthermore, Fall et al. [23] use motion of the shoulders and neck to control the commercially available robot arm JACO [24]. The user can choose between different control modes of JACO to perform 3D-translations, arm and wrist rotations or control the fingers' positions, respectively. The Human–Robot Interface (HRI) presented by Fall et al. requires additional switches to switch between these modes, though.

In our research group, we have developed the AMiCUS system, which is the first interface that uses only head motion to produce all the necessary signals and commands for real-time control of an application with more than three Degrees of Freedom (DOF), such as a robotic arm. Some of the major criteria for the development of such an HRI are the following:

1. The HRI should be adaptive, always using the full available neck range of motion of the user.
2. The relationship between performed head motion and resulting robot motion has to be intuitive.
3. The HRI must reliably distinguish between unintended head motion, head motion intended for direct control and head motion to generate switching commands.
4. The HRI has to give sufficient and useful feedback to the user to allow safe and efficient operation.
5. The HRI must enable the user to perform smooth, precise and efficient robot movements in Cartesian space.
6. The user should enjoy using the HRI.

AMiCUS has been designed with special attention to these requirements. A tetraplegic with severe head motion limitation has been involved in the whole development cycle to ensure the system's relevance for the target group.

In the next section, the hardware, software and signal processing of the resulting system are described. Afterwards, the experimental setup of a user study with 13 able-bodied and 6 tetraplegic subjects to validate the system is presented. Subsequently, the results are presented and discussed. In the last section, these results are compared against aforementioned criteria for a head motion-based HRI.

2. AMiCUS

Within this section we introduce AMiCUS. AMiCUS stands for **A**daptive Head **M**otion **C**ontrol for **U**ser-friendly **S**upport. The demonstrator AMiCUS is the result of several years of research within our research group. First, we will give an overview of our research activities. Then, we describe the sensor placement. This is followed by a description of the used hardware. Next, we present how robot groups have been built in order to control all DOFs of the robot with head motion. Afterwards, the two modes of AMiCUS, namely Robot Control Mode and Cursor Control Mode, are described in detail. The section closes with the presentation of the necessary calibration routines.

2.1. Relation to Previously Published Work

In Reference [25] suitable control modes for real-time control using head motion have been analyzed. Based on the results, a first iteration of the general control structure has been evaluated in References [26,27]. An algorithm to detect head gestures, which can be used as switching commands as part of the chosen control structure has been presented in Reference [28]. Within this work, the whole system that resulted from all previous research is presented and validated in a user study. A usability study of an alternative control structure and GUI for the AMiCUS system has been presented by Jackowski et al. [29]. The system in this publication uses all four head gestures defined in Reference [28] to switch between robot groups, whereas the interface described here uses a control structure based on the work published in References [26,27]. The main advantage of the version presented by Jackowski et al. is that switching between groups is faster, while the main advantage of the version presented here is that it can be used by a wider range of users as explained in detail later in this work.

2.2. Sensor Placement

A MEMS AHRS was chosen to measure the user's head motion. A typical AHRS outputs raw sensor data from a 3D accelerometer, a 3D gyroscope and a 3D magnetometer, as well as sensor orientation obtained from such raw data.

In Reference [30] we showed that a rigid body placed onto a human head is moved on a spherical surface during head motion (Figure 1). For the sake of simplicity, the sensor placement was chosen in a way that the sensor yaw axis and the approximated yaw axis of the user's cervical spine coincided. Given this sensor placement, changes in head and sensor orientation are identical and a transformation of sensor orientation to head orientation is not needed. Nonetheless, an offset calibration remains necessary to define the zero position of the user's head. Every head motion apart from rotation around the yaw-axis results in additional linear sensor movement as the sensor is not rotated around its own center.

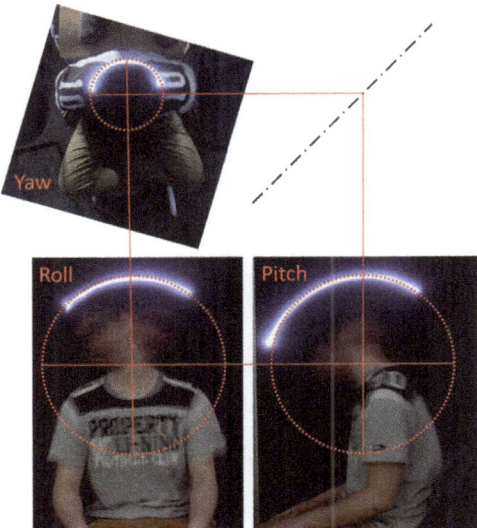

Figure 1. Kinematics of the cervical spine. From the kinematic point of view, the human cervical spine can be approximated by a ball joint. That means, every motion can be divided into single rotations around three orthogonal axes that intersect in one point. This point, that is, the center of rotation, roughly coincides with the location of the thyroid gland. As a result, a rigid body placed onto a human head moves on a spherical surface during head motion.

2.3. Hardware

AMiCUS detects head motion using a Hillcrest FSM-9 motion sensor system [31], which is placed as described in the previous section. Output data of the sensor system under static conditions and during head motion are provided in the Supplementary Materials. The acquired sensor data is processed on a desktop computer with the AMiCUS software, which is written in C++ using the Qt framework [32]. The resulting control signals are transmitted to a Universal Robots UR5 robot arm [33] which is equipped with a Robotiq 2-Finger parallel gripper [34]. By default, the position of the gripper can be controlled in world coordinates ${}^{w}\mathbf{p} = {}^{w}(x,y,z)^T$ as well as gripper coordinates ${}^{g}\mathbf{p} = {}^{g}(x,y,z)^T$ using inverse kinematics. These coordinate systems are shown in Figure 2. Rotations of the gripper are performed in gripper coordinates ${}^{g}\boldsymbol{\alpha} = {}^{g}(\varphi, \vartheta, \psi)^T$. The gripper can be opened and closed in order to interact with objects. The position of the gripper's fingers is denoted as β. All these DOFs, ${}^{r}\mathbf{s} = \left({}^{w/g}\mathbf{p}, {}^{g}\boldsymbol{\alpha}, \beta\right)^T$, can be controlled proportionally. That means that the signal amplitude can be varied continuously. A Logitech C930e webcam [35] is mounted on the gripper to provide feedback during positioning and gripping. The camera image is part of the Graphical User Interface (GUI) of AMiCUS. The GUI is displayed on an ordinary computer screen in front of the user.

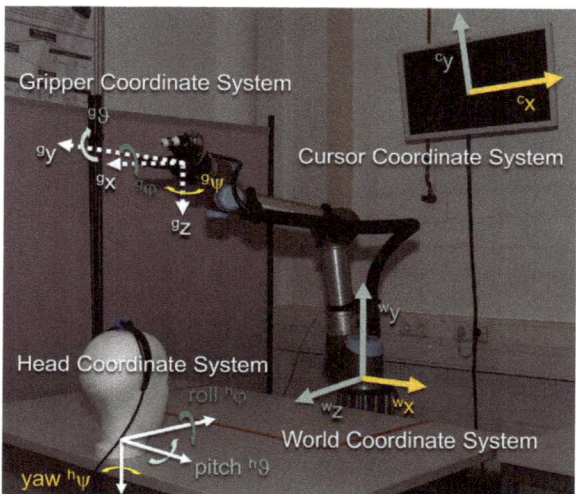

Figure 2. Coordinate systems of the AMiCUS system. Degrees of Freedom (DOFs) of the same color are controlled by the same head DOF. The zero orientation of the head coordinate system depends on whether the cursor or the robot is controlled. During robot control, the head coordinate system is denoted by ${}^{h_r}\boldsymbol{\alpha} = {}^{h_r}(\varphi, \vartheta, \psi)^T$ and ${}^{h_c}\boldsymbol{\alpha} = {}^{h_c}(\varphi, \vartheta, \psi)^T$ during cursor control.

2.4. Robot Groups

Three proportional control signals are provided through head motion, that is, ${}^{h}\boldsymbol{\alpha} = {}^{h}(\varphi, \vartheta, \psi)^T$. With these signals, seven DOFs of the robot, ${}^{r}\mathbf{s}$, have to be controlled. That means, direct robot control in terms of a 1:1-mapping is not feasible. For this reason, groups containing maximum three DOFs of the robot have been defined, namely Gripper, Vertical Plane, Horizontal Plane and Orientation. The DOFs of the head have been mapped onto the DOFs of the robot as follows (Figure 3):

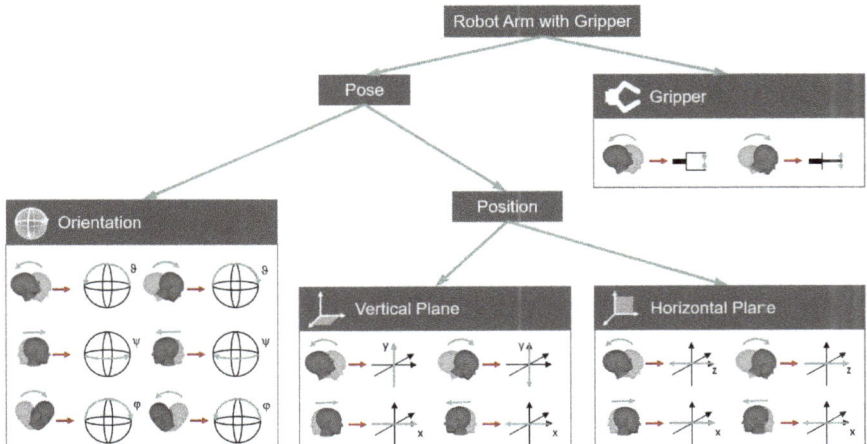

Figure 3. Mapping of head DOFs onto robot DOFs. Four different groups, that is, Gripper, Orientation, Vertical Plane and Horizontal Plane, are depicted. The user is able to switch between groups in order to control all DOFs of the robot.

In the Gripper group, the gripper can be opened and closed using the pitch motion of the user's head ($^h\vartheta \mapsto \beta$). The group Vertical Plane enables the user to move the gripper within a plane that is perpendicular to the user's line of sight. The user can move the gripper to the left or right by turning the head to the left or right ($^h\psi \mapsto {^w}x$). In order to move the gripper up or down, one has to tilt the head up or down ($^h\vartheta \mapsto {^w}y$). The gripper can be moved back or forth in the Horizontal Plane group by tilting the head down or up ($^h\vartheta \mapsto {^w}z$). Additionally, the user can move the robot left and right the same way as in the Vertical Plane group.

The orientation of the gripper is controlled in the Orientation group. Each rotary movement of the head is mapped onto the corresponding rotation of the gripper. That means, the roll rotation of the gripper is controlled by the roll rotation of the head ($^h\varphi \mapsto {^g}\varphi$); the control of the pitch rotation of the gripper is performed using the pitch rotation of the head ($^h\vartheta \mapsto {^g}\vartheta$); and the yaw rotation of the gripper is controlled by the yaw rotation of the head ($^h\psi \mapsto {^g}\psi$).

2.5. Robot Control Mode

During direct robot control within one of the robot groups, the position along a head DOF is projected onto the velocity along a robot DOF ($\gamma \mapsto \dot{g}$), with $\gamma \in {^h}\boldsymbol{\alpha}$ and $g \in {^r}\mathbf{s}$ [25].

A GOMPERTZ-function is used as the transfer function (Figure 4). Using this function, head motion close to zero position, which is likely to be unintended, is not translated into robot motion (Deadzone). If the user keeps increasing head deflection, the robot slowly starts to move into the desired direction. Small deflection angles of the head enable slow, precise robot control. An increase of head deflection leads to an exceedingly smooth transition to fast, imprecise robot control. Mathmatically, the implemented transfer function can be formulated as:

$$\dot{g} = \begin{cases} A_{\max} \cdot e^{\delta \cdot e^{r \cdot \gamma_n}} & \text{if } \gamma > 0 \\ -A_{\max} \cdot e^{\delta \cdot e^{-r \cdot \gamma_n}} & \text{else} \end{cases} \tag{1a}$$

$$\gamma_n = \frac{\gamma}{\gamma_{\text{th}}} \tag{1b}$$

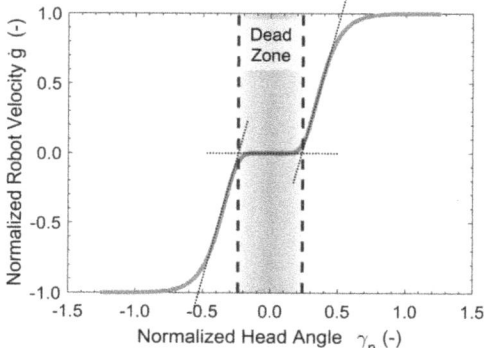

Figure 4. Robot control transfer function. A GOMPERTZ-function is used as transfer function. The used parameters are $A_{max} = 1$, $\delta = -30$ and $r = -10$. The space between the dashed lines indicates the deadzone.

The parameter $A_{max} \in \mathbb{R}^+$ indicates the upper asymptote. This corresponds to maximum velocity in g-direction. The coefficient $\delta \in \mathbb{R}^-$ sets the displacements along the γ-axis and $r \in \mathbb{R}^-$ indicates the growth rate. The parameters δ and r are identical for all the robot DOFs. The amplitude A_{max} is adjusted separately for the linear DOFs $^w\mathbf{p}$, the rotational DOFs $^g\boldsymbol{\alpha}$ and the gripper β. The parameter γ_{th} defines the range of motion along the γ-axis, which shall be used for control. This range as well as the zero position are obtained during a calibration routine as described later.

For every time step of length Δt, the new robot state $^r\mathbf{s}_{new}$ is computed using the following relationship:

$$^r\mathbf{s}_{new} = {}^r\mathbf{s}_{old} + {}^r\dot{\mathbf{s}} \cdot \Delta t \qquad (2)$$

If the linear acceleration of the sensor during control exceeds a certain threshold, robot control is deactivated. This is supposed to guarantee operational safety as quick movements are likely to not be intended for robot control. After deactiviation, the user has to turn his head to the zero position in order to continue control. This event is accompanied by visual and acoustic feedback.

The normalized head angles γ_n are displayed in real-time on the GUI during Robot Control Mode. Additionally, a picture of the current robot group and the image of the gripper camera are shown (Figure 5).

During Robot Control Mode, all DOFs of the chosen group can be controlled simultaneously. However, switching is necessary to control the DOFs of another group. The user can leave the current group by performing a Head Gesture, which is described in the following.

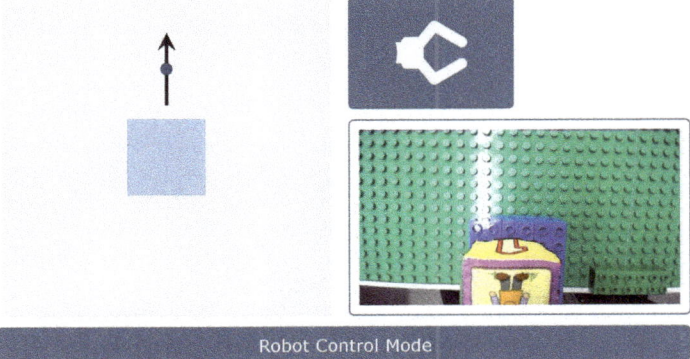

Figure 5. Graphical User Interface during Robot Control Mode. The GUI displays an icon of the current robot group (top right), the image of the gripper camera (bottom right), an information line (bottom) and feedback about the current head angle given by the arrow (left). The square represents the deadzone in which the robot arm cannot be moved.

Head Gesture

The Head Gesture denotes a nodding-like movement (Figure 6). More precisely, the user has to quickly move the head down starting from zero position and back. Mathematically, the shape of the gesture can be described by a Gaussian function:

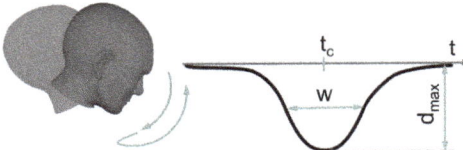

Figure 6. Head Gesture. The gesture is displayed with its $^{h_r}\vartheta$-angles over time t. Parameters: d_{max} = amplitude, w = peak width, t_c = location of the peak center.

$$d = d_{max} \cdot e^{-\left(\frac{t-t_c}{w}\right)^2} \tag{3}$$

Maximum head displacement is expressed by the amplitude d_{max}, t_c is the centroid and w is related to the peak width. The implemented algorithm for robust Head Gesture recognition in a real-time data stream has been presented in Reference [28]. Briefly summarized, the algorithm assumes that activity is present when the magnitude of linear acceleration of the sensor exceeds a certain threshold. If activity is present, both head angles $^{h_r}\alpha$ and sensor data are recorded. Recording stops when activity is no longer present. If the length of the recorded data lies between 0.25 s and 2 s and the dominating initial linear acceleration has been in positive ^{h}x-direction (Figure 2), the recorded data might contain a Head Gesture. For validation, a Gaussian function is fitted to the recorded $^{h_r}\vartheta$-angles. The Head Gesture is classified if the following conditions are fulfilled:

- The neck was flexed sufficiently ($d_{max} < -20°$).
- The gesture was performed quickly enough ($w < 0.4$ s).
- The gesture was suffiently Gaussian-shaped ($R^2 > 0.75$).
- The maximum $^{h_r}\varphi$- and $^{h_r}\psi$-angles did not exceed 80 % of $|d_{max}|$

In case the Head Gesture has not been performed correctly, visual feedback is shown on the GUI that informs the user how to adjust a movement for successful Head Gesture detection. In case of correct gesture execution, the system switches from Robot Control Mode to Cursor Control Mode.

2.6. Cursor Control Mode

During Cursor Control Mode, the user controls a mouse cursor on the GUI using head motion to select a different robot group or to perform any other action, such as starting a calibration routine or pausing control.

To control the mouse cursor, the user's head orientation is directly mapped onto the position of the cursor [25]. That means, the pitch-DOF is mapped linearly onto the $^c y$-axis of the screen ($^h\vartheta \mapsto {}^c y$), while the yaw-DOF is mapped onto the $^c x$-axis of the screen ($^h\psi \mapsto {}^c x$). This relationship is described by:

$$^c\mathbf{s} = \begin{pmatrix} ^c x \\ ^c y \end{pmatrix} = \operatorname{diag}\left(^h_c\mathbf{m}\right) \cdot \begin{pmatrix} ^h\psi \\ ^h\vartheta \end{pmatrix} + {}^c\mathbf{b} \qquad (4)$$

The parameters $^h_c\mathbf{m} = {}^h_c(m_x, m_y)^T$ reflect the sensitivity. The parameters $^c\mathbf{b} = {}^c(b_x, b_y)^T$ indicate the cursor coordinates when the head is in its zero position, $^{hc}(\vartheta, \psi)_0^T$. The corresponding values are obtained during a later described calibration routine.

By moving the mouse cursor, the user interacts with the GUI that is shown during Cursor Control Mode (Cursor GUI, Figure 7). This GUI contains dwell buttons, for example, to start the calibration routines, pause control, switch between coordinate systems or close the program. A dwell button is activated by dwelling on it for 2 s. In addition to the dwell buttons, the GUI contains a Slide Button for each robot group. A robot group is selected by activating the corresponding Slide Button.

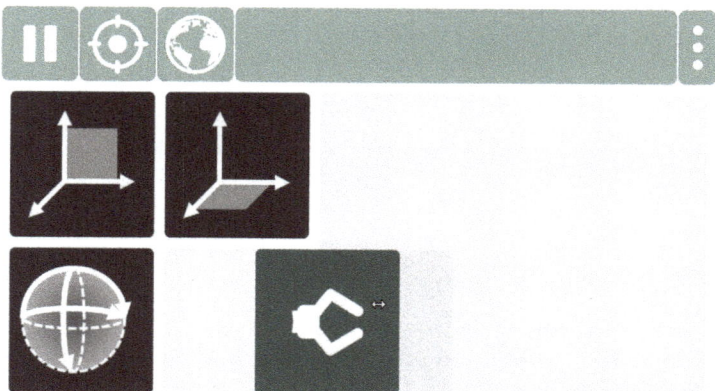

Figure 7. Graphical User Interface during Cursor Control Mode. The GUI contains one Slide Button for each robot group. The dwell buttons in the top toolbar allow the user to perform several actions, such as pausing control, starting calibration routines or exiting the program.

Slide Button

For successful activation of the Slide Button, the following steps are necessary (Figure 8): First, the user has to hover the Slide Button with the mouse cursor and dwell there for a certain time (State 1). Then, a rail rolls out in order to inform the user that the button can be slid to the right as indicated by the rail (State 2). If the cursor is moved to the right in a straight line, the Slide Button moves with it. If the user leaves the Slide Button area by moving the cursor up, down or left, the action is immediately aborted. After sliding the button to the right end of the rail (State 3), the user has to move the Slide

Button back to the left. The action is aborted when leaving the Slide Button area to the top, bottom or right. If the Slide Button is moved to the left along the rail correctly, the rail rolls up and the robot group associated with the Slide Button is entered. Each state of the Slide Button is accompanied by visual and acoustic feedback.

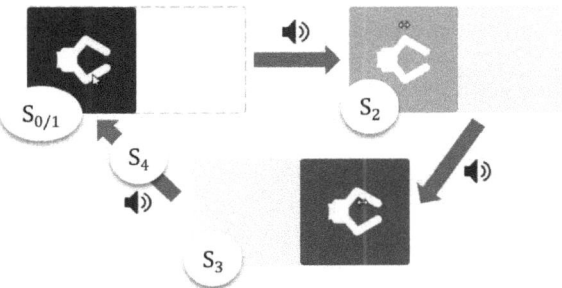

Figure 8. Slide Button. The following steps are necessary for successful activation: When the button is in its neutral state (S_0) the mouse cursor has to dwell in the button (S_1) until visual and acoustic feedback occurs. Then, the button has to be moved to the right along the rail (S_2). At the end of the rail visual and acoustic feedback is given. Next, the button has to be moved to the left along the rail (S_3). When the button reaches the initial position (S_4), it is activated and the assigned action is performed.

2.7. Calibration Routines

2.7.1. Robot Calibration

The calibration routine, which is needed to control the robot arm during Robot Control Mode, is called Robot Calibration. At the beginning of the Robot Calibration, the user has to define the zero position of the head coordinate system, ${}^{hr}\pmb{\alpha}_0$. The zero position should be chosen in a way that the user faces the robot arm. This position has to be held for 2 s within a tolerance of $2°$. Afterwards, the corresponding Euler angles of the sensor are saved as offset ${}^s\pmb{\alpha}_{0,r} = {}^s(\varphi, \vartheta, \psi)_{0,r}^T$. The offset is subtracted from the sensor angles ${}^s\pmb{\alpha}$ in order to obtain head angles ${}^{hr}\pmb{\alpha}$.

After offset definition, the user has to perform each one repetition of neck flexion and extension, neck lateral bending to the left and to the right and neck rotation to the left and to the right. Pictures of these positions are displayed on the GUI. The users are instructed to move their heads as far as they can while still being able to see the robot. After holding a certain position, the corresponding head angle of the relevant DOF is saved and the next position is displayed. In this way two values are obtained for each DOF: One in positive direction (γ_+) and one in negative one (γ_-). To guarantee a symmetrical mapping, only the smaller value is used to define the range of motion γ_{th}.

Whenever a calibration point is saved, acoustic feedback is given to the user. Furthermore, a status bar indicates how long the user has to hold the head stable until a calibration point is saved.

2.7.2. Cursor Calibration

The calibration that is necessary to control the mouse cursor during Cursor Control Mode is denoted as Cursor Calibration. During Cursor Calibration, the user has to turn the head towards five targets, which are shown on the screen one after the other. A calibration point is saved when the user holds the head stable for 2 s within a tolerance of $2°$. The first target is shown in the center of the screen. The user's head orientation when facing this point is defined as the zero position of the head during cursor control, ${}^{hc}(\vartheta, \psi)_0^T$. The corresponding sensor angles ${}^s(\vartheta, \psi)_{0,c}^T$ are defined as the offset between the head and the sensor coordinate system. For all samples, the offset is subtracted from the sensor angles ${}^s(\vartheta, \psi)^T$ to obtain the head coordinates ${}^{hc}(\vartheta, \psi)^T$ explicitly. This step ensures that Gimbal Lock does not occur. For every target, the head angles ${}^{hc}(\vartheta, \psi)^T$ and the position of the target on the screen

^{c}**s** are saved. The remaining targets are displayed in the upper left corner, center, lower right corner and in the center again. Whenever a calibration point is saved, acoustic feedback is given. At the end of the calibration procedure, the parameters $^h_c\mathbf{m}$ and $^c\mathbf{b}$ are computed from the five calibration points using a minimum least squares fit. Head angles corresponding to the center of the screen are acquired three times to obtain more reliable data for this point. This is important, because the correct calibration of the center point has a major impact on the subjective calibration success perceived by the user.

3. Materials and Methods

The aim of the study was providing a proof-of-concept of the AMiCUS system. That means, showing that AMiCUS enabled people to perform simple manipulation tasks with the robot arm efficiently. Furthermore, we wanted to investigate if all aforementioned criteria for a head motion-based HRI were met and at which points AMiCUS could be developed further.

3.1. Subjects

Thirteen able-bodied subjects and six teraplegics took part in the experiments. The able-bodied subjects were recruited via announcements on the university website and in the local newspapers. Six of them were male, seven female. Their mean age was 37.0 ± 15.0 years. The able-bodied subjects had no known neck motion limitations and carried out the experiments at the Westphalian University of Applied Sciences in Gelsenkirchen. The able-bodied subjects represented users with full Range of Motion (full ROM).

The tetraplegics were recruited via the BG-Hospital Hamburg where they also carried out the experiments. Five of them were male, one female. Their mean age was 35.7 ± 15.2 years. The levels of injury ranged from C0 to C4. Subjects with both complete and incomplete injuries were included. The tetraplegics were chosen to have severe neck motion limitations in order to represent users with restricted Range of Motion (restricted ROM). It is worth noting that all of these tetraplegics were unable to operate the system presented in Reference [29] due to their neck motion limitations.

None of the subjects had prior experience with AMiCUS. The study was approved by the ethics committee of the University of Bremen and the subjects gave their informed consent prior to participation.

3.2. Experimental Setup

The subjects were seated in front of a table with an arrangement of platforms and softcubes according to the particular task to be performed. The robot arm was positioned on the opposite side of the table, facing the current subject.

The GUI was displayed on a 27″ screen, which was mounted behind the robot arm. The horizontal distance of the screen from the subject was approximately 2.4 m. The screen was positioned in a way that it was not occluded by the robot. Small deviations between the experimental setups for the able-bodied and tetraplegic subjects could not be avoided due to different spatial conditions.

The used sensor settings are shown in Table 1. The sampling rate for the raw and fused sensor data was set to 125 Hz. This is the recommended minimum sample rate for the sensor fusion algorithm to work properly. The accuracy of the orientation output was specified as $1.5°$ by the manufacturer. The sensor data was downsampled to 60 Hz for further processing to save computing power while still displaying head orientation smoothly on the screen. The calculation of the joint angles using inverse kinematics and the physical robot movement needed almost 0.04 s. For this reason, the 60 Hz control signals to update the robot's joint angles were further downsampled to 25 Hz.

Both the linear acceleration and angular position output were used for the gesture recognition. The data was processed as described in Reference [28]. The control signals for the cursor and robot arm were generated based on the angular position output as described in Section 2.

Table 1. Settings of the Hillcrest FSM-9.

Setting	Value	Meaning
Samplerate	125 Hz	
Operating Mode	4	Full Motion on
Packet Select	8	Motion Engine output
Format Select	0	Format 0 packet
FF2	true	Enable output of linear acceleration, no gravity
FF6	true	Enable output of angular position

3.3. Procedure

A trial session, a predefined task and a complex task were part of the experimental study. The procedure was identical to the usability study performed with the alternative AMiCUS version as described in Reference [29]. This was done to allow for a better comparison of both versions. However, such a comparison is beyond the scope of the work presented here.

3.3.1. Trial Session

Prior to the trial session, the subjects were shown an introduction video that demonstrated the basic working principle and modes of operation of AMiCUS. Video instructions were chosen to make sure every subject received the same information. After the video, the subjects were free to try the system for 10 min. They were encouraged to enter each robot group at least once.

3.3.2. Predefined Task

After completing the trial session, a video of the predefined task was shown. For the tasks, five square-shaped platforms with 9.5 cm edge length and three softcubes with 6.5 cm edge length were arranged as shown in Figure 9.

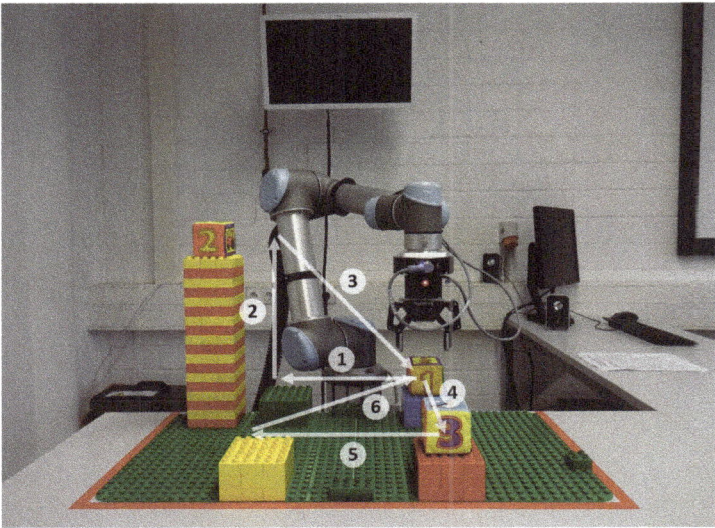

Figure 9. Experimental setup of the predefined task. The subjects were clearly instructed how to move the robot. Movements 1–3 had to be performed in the Vertical Plane group, movements 4–6 in the Horizontal Plane group. After movement 6, the subjects had to perform one 90°-rotation around each rotation axis.

First, cube 1 had to be moved from the blue to the green platform (1). After placing the cube on the green platform, the gripper had to be moved to the top of the tower (2) to grip cube 2 and move it to the blue platform (3). Afterwards, the gripper had to be moved to the red platform (4) and cube 3 had to be transported to the yellow platform (5). Finally, the gripper had to be moved to the blue platform (6). After arriving at the blue platform, cube 1 had to be gripped, lifted a little bit and rotated around 90° in positive $^g\vartheta$-direction, then around 90° in negative $^g\psi$-direction and finally around 90° in positive $^g\varphi$-direction.

In order to solve this task, all subjects received detailed instructions about the desired control steps to be performed. Movements 1–3 had to be performed in the Vertical Plane group, movements 4–6 in the Horizontal Plane group and the rotations in the Orientation group.

3.3.3. Complex Task

During the complex task, 3 softcubes were placed on a table as shown in Figure 10a. The users were told to stack the cubes on top of each other in a way that softcube 1 was on the formerly empty platform, softcube 2 in the middle and softcube 3 on top of the stack. In addition, a picture of the solution has been shown to the subjects prior to the task (Figure 10b). The subjects had to find their own control strategy to solve the task.

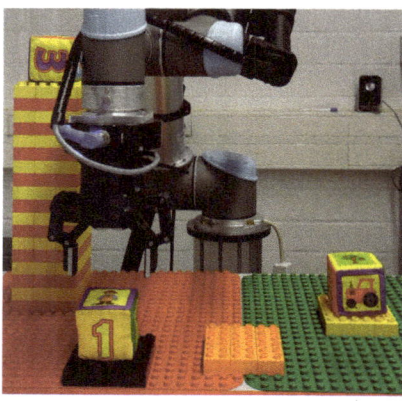 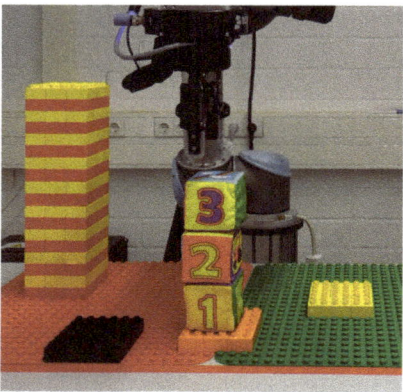

(a) Initial setup   (b) Target setup

Figure 10. Experimental setup of the complex task. The users had to find their own control strategy to solve the task.

3.4. Evaluation Criteria

3.4.1. Objective Evaluation

The completion rates were obtained for both the predefined and complex task. Subjects had only one trial to complete the tasks. A task was counted as failed when manual assistance from the experimenters was needed to proceed, when the subjects used their hands or when the task was executed incorrectly. Completion time was considered unsuitable as an evaluation criterion because of too many disturbing influences, for example, due to talking.

For both the Slide Button and the Head Gesture success rate and activation time were chosen as evaluation criteria. Success rate was evaluated using data of both the predefined and the complex task, whereas activation time contained only data from the predefined task. Activation time was defined as the time from the spoken command of the experimenter until the change of mode was visible on the GUI. That means that failed attempts were also included in the activation time. As a result, activation time and success rate are correlated. The medians of the activation times and success rates were first computed subject-wise. Based on these data, medians and quartiles were obtained for all subjects together. Differences between Slide Button and Head Gesture were evaluated utilizing paired-sample t-tests [36]. An overview of statistical tests can be found in Reference [37].

3.4.2. Subjective Evaluation

For the subjective evaluation of the system, all subjects completed an evaluation sheet. This sheet contained 30 statements, regarding calibration, GUI, switching, mapping, transfer function and general aspects, which could be rated between 1 (*"I strongly disagree"*) and 5 (*"I strongly agree"*) (Table 2). Three additional statements regarding the speed of operation could be rated between 1 (*"Far too slow"*) and 5 (*"Far too fast"*). The answers were compared with each other using Friedman's tests [38]. The significance level for the tests was 5 %.

4. Results and Discussion

4.1. Objective Evaluation

4.1.1. Completion Rates

All subjects, independent of available range of motion, were able to get a general understanding of the control structure and could move the robot arm in a controlled manner, as demonstrated in the trial session. It is worth mentioning that all subjects were first-time users of AMiCUS and did not have prior experience with any other head-controlled system.

The Fisher's exact test [39] indicated that there was no significant difference between the users with full and restricted ROM regarding task completion rates. Therefore, the completion rates are presented for all subjects together. All subjects were able to complete the predefined task, resulting in a completion rate of 100 %. The overall completion rate of the complex task was 72.2 % (Figure 11). In 16.7 % of the cases, manual assistance was required to solve the task at all or within a reasonable time period. In each 5.6 % of the cases, hand-use or stack-collapse led to task failure. It is notable, that 60 % of the non-completions resulted from inaccurate gripper positioning in $^w z$-direction.

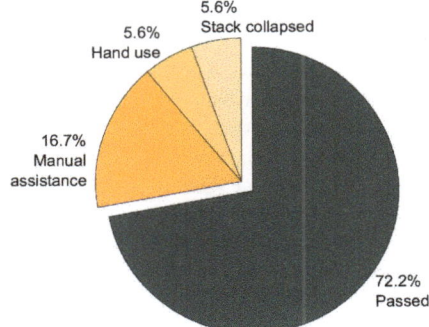

Figure 11. Completion rate of the complex task. There was no statistical difference between the users with full and restricted ROM. The overall completion rate of the complex task was 72.2 % (n = 18).

4.1.2. Success Rates and Activation Times

The success rate of the Slide Button was 85.80 % for the subjects with full ROM (Figure 12a). For the subjects with restricted ROM it was 82.52 %. When the first attempt failed, the subjects with full ROM activated the Slide Button successfully after the second attempt in 12.60 % of the cases. The subjects with restricted ROM succeeded after the second attempt in 14.23 %. In 1.32 %, the subjects with full ROM needed three attempts to successfully activate the Slide Button. The subjects with restricted ROM needed three attempts in 3.25 % of the cases. In the remaining 0.28 %, more than three attempts were needed by the subjects with full ROM. The subjects with restricted ROM did not need more than three attempts.

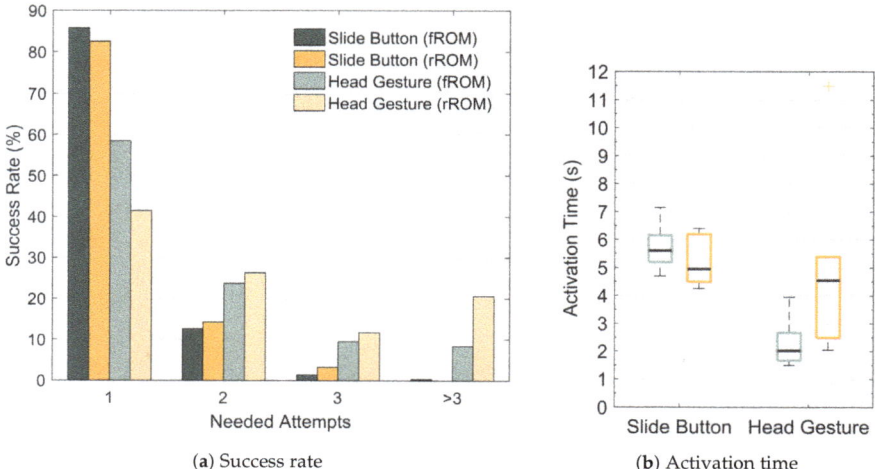

Figure 12. Comparison between Slide Button and Head Gesture. The performance of the Slide Button and the Head Gesture was evaluated in terms of success rate and activation time.

In Figure 12b the activation times for the Slide Button and for the Head Gesture are shown based on the median activation times for each subject. For the Slide Button the median activation time was 5.6 s for the subjects with full ROM and 5.0 s for the subjects with restricted ROM. The two-sample t-test [36] indicated no significant difference between both groups. However, for the subjects with full ROM the median activation time of the Head Gesture was 2.0 s. This is almost three times faster than the Slide Button activation, even though all failed activation attempts were included in the activation time. This difference is significant. For the subjects with restricted ROM the median activation time of the Head Gesture was 4.6 s. That means, the subjects with restricted ROM needed significantly more time to perform the Head Gesture correctly than the subjects with full ROM (two-sample t-test). Futhermore, according to a paired-sample t-test, the activation times of the Head Gesture and the Slide Button did not differ significantly for the subjects with restricted ROM.

It is important to note that the execution time for a single Head Gesture had to lie between 0.25 s and 2 s. Movements beyond these bounds were not taken into account by the classification algorithm. That means that a certain execution speed was enforced for the Head Gesture while the Slide Button could be moved as slowly as desired. The fact that the Head Gesture had to be performed both quickly and accurately led to a significant lower success rate of the Head Gesture compared to the Slide Button for both groups (paired-sample t-tests): The success rate of the Head Gesture for the subjects with full ROM was 58.45 % and 41.45 % for the subjects with restricted ROM. In 23.68 % of all cases, the second attempt was successful for the subjects with full ROM. The subjects with restricted ROM succeeded after the second attempt in 26.27 % of all cases. Three attempts were needed by the subjects with full ROM in 9.51 % of all cases. The subjects with restricted ROM performed the Head Gesture correctly after the third attempt in 11.69 % of the cases. In 8.36 % of the cases more than three attempts were needed by the subjects with full ROM, while the subjects with restricted ROM needed more than three attempts in 20.59 % of the cases. It is notable that the maximum number of observed failed attempts was 16 for the Head Gesture while it was 4 for the Slide Button. Though the non-detection rate of the gesture was relatively high, the robot did not move unintendedly, which is very important from a safety point of view.

In conclusion, for both groups the success rate of the Head Gesture was significantly lower than the one of the Slide Button. On the other hand, the activation time of the Head Gesture was significantly lower for the subjects with full ROM. However, this difference was not present for the subjects with restricted ROM: The results indicate that the correct execution of the Head Gesture becomes more difficult when the ROM is restricted, while based on our results, the level of difficulty of the Slide Button is not affected significantly by the available ROM of the user.

4.2. Subjective Evaluation

The Mann-Whitney U-test [40] indicated no significant differences between the subjects with full and restricted ROM. Hence, the ratings from both groups have been assumed to originate from the same distribution and are therefore presented together.

Table 2. Evaluation sheet for AMiCUS including results.

Topic	No.	Statement	Rating
Calibration	1	Understanding what one is supposed to do during Cursor Calibration is easy	4.83 ± 0.38
	2	Understanding what one is supposed to do during Robot Calibration is easy	4.81 ± 0.40
	3	The acoustic feedback during calibration is useful	4.88 ± 0.33
GUI	4	The Cursor GUI is visually appealing and clearly structured	4.39 ± 0.61
	5	In Cursor Mode, all important functions can be accessed easily	4.61 ± 0.61
	6	The Robot GUI is visually appealing and clearly structured	4.33 ± 0.69
	7	In Robot Mode, all important information is displayed on the GUI	4.41 ± 0.71
	8	The feedback about the current head position is easy to understand and useful	4.78 ± 0.43
	9	The camera image is useful	4.33 ± 1.14
Switching	10	Activating the Slide Button is easy	4.56 ± 0.62
	11	The acoustic and visual feedback for the Slide Button is useful	4.44 ± 0.92
	12	Performing the Head Gesture correctly is easy	3.33 ± 1.46
	13	The feedback about Head Gesture execution is useful	3.89 ± 1.37
	14	Switching between groups is easy	4.06 ± 0.94
	15	Switching between groups is quick	3.33 ± 0.91
Mapping	16	I can well imagine what the gripper does when I move my head up or down	4.61 ± 0.78
	17	I can well imagine what the robot does in Vertical Plane group when I move my head up or down	4.72 ± 0.75
	18	I can well imagine what the robot does in Vertical Plane or Horizontal Plane group when I turn my head to the left or to the right	4.56 ± 0.86
	19	I can well imagine what the robot does in Horizontal Plane group when I move my head up or down	4.28 ± 1.02
	20	I can well imagine what the robot does in Orientation group when I move my head up or down	3.44 ± 1.25
	21	I can well imagine what the robot does in Orientation group when I turn my head to the left or to the right	3.44 ± 1.15
	22	I can well imagine what the robot does in Orientation group when I bend my head to the left or to the right	3.33 ± 1.24
Transfer function	23	Moving the mouse cursor precisely is easy	4.44 ± 0.62
	24	Gripping precisely is easy	4.17 ± 1.15
	25	Moving the robot arm precisely is easy	4.44 ± 0.70
General	26	Assessing robot position correctly in Vertical Plane group is easy	4.56 ± 0.70
	27	Assessing robot position correctly in Horizontal Plane group is easy	4.28 ± 0.75
	28	Assessing robot orientation correctly is easy	2.89 ± 1.18
	29	I can easily keep an eye an all relevant parts of the system	3.94 ± 1.26
	30	Robot control is fun	4.72 ± 0.46

Rating: 1 = "I strongly disagree", 2 = "I disagree", 3 = "I partly agree", 4 = "I agree", 5 = "I strongly agree".

4.2.1. Calibration

As Table 2 shows, the majority of subjects found both the Cursor as well as the Robot Calibration highly intuitive. Furthermore, the acoustic feedback to indicate that a calibration point has been saved was perceived as very useful.

4.2.2. GUI

The subjects considered both the Cursor GUI and the Robot GUI visually appealing and clearly structured. They agreed that all important functions were easily accessible during cursor control. Moreover, the majority of subjects had the opinion that all important information was displayed on the GUI during robot control. A few subjects remarked that more information could be helpful. The feedback showing the current head orientation was experienced as very useful. The camera image was mainly considered useful, even though a few subjects remarked that they had not paid much attention to the camera image during control. This is likely, because it was not mandatory for the given tasks. However, there are scenarios in which the gripper camera is necessary because direct view is obstructed.

4.2.3. Switching

The Slide Button activation was rated very easy. This is also in line with the high success rate of the Slide Button. The vast majority of the subjects perceived the acoustic and visual feedback of the Slide Button as useful or very useful but some subjects found the acoustic feedback disturbing after a while. The Head Gesture has been found to be significantly more difficult than the Slide Button. This is also represented by the lower success rate of the Head Gesture. Some subjects remarked that they perceived the Head Gesture as a stress-inducing factor. Observations during the experiments indicate that the gesture execution was demanding for some subjects with restricted ROM. The entire switching procedure was mainly rated as easy. Most subjects rated switching between groups as too slow. The common opinion was that the Head Gesture and also the Slide Button alone were quick enough but the combination was not. All in all, the Head Gesture was not considered easy to execute and the associated feedback was not considered helpful.

4.2.4. Mapping

In order to evaluate the intuitiveness of the mapping, the subjects were asked how well they could imagine how the robot would respond to their head motion. The results indicate that the subjects found it highly intuitive to open or close the gripper using pitch motion. Furthermore, they strongly agreed that they could well imagine that the robot moved up or down in the Vertical Plane group when they tilted their heads up or down. The majority of the subjects could also imagine well how the robot would move if they rotated their heads left or right. Most subjects agreed that they could imagine well how the robot would move in the Horizontal Plane group when they tilted their heads up or down. However, the vast majority remarked that they would have found it more intuitive if the direction of the robot motion had been switched, that is, that the robot moved closer to the subjects when they tilted their heads down and vice versa. This is also in line with the observation that many subjects initially moved the robot in the wrong direction during movements 4 and 6 of the predefined task. The intuitiveness of the mapping for the DOFs of the Orientation group was significantly lower than for the DOFs of the Vertical Plane group or the Gripper. The subjects criticized that they found it hard to imagine rotations in local coordinates of the gripper. But they agreed that it became a lot easier after they had been instructed to imagine the gripper to have a face with the camera as the eyes and the gripper as the mouth. A possible explanation is that the gripper movements may then be processed in different parts of the brain, such as the Fusiform Face Area. Once the gripper is interpreted as a face, mirror neurons may map its movements onto the subjects' own head movements.

4.2.5. Transfer Function

The majority of subjects strongly agreed that it was very easy to move the mouse cursor precisely under the testing conditions. This is in line with the high success rate of the Slide Button. Furthermore, the subjects found precise positioning of the mouse cursor significantly easier than gripping or moving the robot arm precisely. A few subjects annotated that they found the mouse cursor too fast. This problem can be solved by decreasing the distance between subject and screen or by choosing a larger screen. Gripping accurately was mainly considered as easy. Some subjects criticized that the gripper could not be opened and closed smoothly. This problem was caused by the gripper and can only be solved by changing the gripper hardware. On average, subjects agreed that accurate positioning of the robot arm was easy. The subjects who partly agreed to that statement mainly argued that they sometimes lacked feedback for accurate positioning. Nonetheless, all the subjects were able to complete the tasks without colliding. The velocities for opening/closing the gripper, linear motion and rotational motion have been assessed suitable by almost all subjects (Figure 13). More experienced users might find robot control too slow. However, the AMiCUS system allows the adjustment of maximum robot velocity.

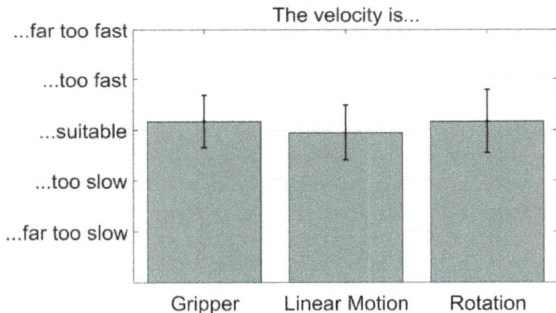

Figure 13. Control speed evaluation. Mean and standard deviation of subjective velocities during gripping, linear motion and rotations (n = 18).

4.2.6. General

The majority of subjects found it easy or very easy to assess robot position correctly in both the Vertical Plane and Horizontal Plane group. However, some subjects asked for additional feedback for accurate positioning. Assessing robot orientation correctly was experienced as significantly more difficult than assessing robot position. Most subjects had no problems with attention loss when looking back and forth between screen, robot and test course. In general, the system has been greatly accepted by the subjects: All of them found that robot control with AMiCUS was fun.

5. Conclusions

Within this work, we presented the AMiCUS system and evaluated it in a user study with 13 able-bodied and 6 tetraplegic subjects. In this section, we validate that the requirements are met and we compare the system presented here with previously published work.

5.1. Compliance with Requirements for a Head Motion-Based HRI

In the following, we step through the list of criteria for a solely head motion-based HRI in order to validate that all requirements are met:

1. The HRI should be adaptive, always using the full available neck range of motion of the user.

During the calibration routine, AMiCUS is adapted to the available neck range of motion of the user. Possible constraints are only imposed by required head gestures. For our experiments, 6 tetraplegics have been recruited that were unable to operate the AMiCUS version in Reference [29] due to severe head motion limitations that restricted their ability to perform head gestures. All of these subjects were able to successfully operate the robot arm with the version presented here. This makes our version available for a wider range of users. Furthermore, the control structure here can easily be adapted to users that can only use one or two head DOFs by introducing more robot groups with fewer DOFs in the mapping.

2. The relationship between performed head motion and resulting robot motion has to be intuitive.

In general, the relationship between performed head motion and resulting robot motion is intuitive, as all first-time users were able to operate the robot arm. However, further improvements are still possible: The direction of the mapping onto the $^w z$-axis should be inverted in the future. That means, the robot should move closer to the user when turning the head down and further away when turning the head up. Moreover, performing rotations was generally considered as challenging. This resulted mainly from the fact that subjects found it difficult to imagine rotations in gripper coordinates. However, after they were instructed to imagine the gripper as a face, they perceived rotations as easier. In order to facilitate the interpretation of the gripper as a head, the design of the gripper including the camera may be adapted in a way that the gripper resembles a face more. Further attempts to increase intuitiveness may also focus on performing rotations in world coordinates instead of gripper coordinates. Additionally, future versions of AMiCUS may include an option to disable simultaneous rotations because the vast majority of subjects was confused by coupled rotations. However, observations in our research group strongly indicate that rotations in local coordinates as well as simultaneous rotations are not an issue for more experienced users.

3. The HRI must reliably distinguish between unintended head motion, head motion intended for direct control and head motion to generate switching commands.

It could be demonstrated that the robot did not move unintendedly. That means, AMiCUS could reliably distinguish between head motion intended for robot control and head gestures or unintended head motion. Furthermore, unintended head motion has never been classified as a switching command. These facts give a positive prognosis for safety requirements of a possible product implementation. However, in some cases head motion intended to perform a Head Gesture or Slide Button activation has not been detected because the head movements have not been performed as defined. Given these inevitable imperfections of the user to perform head movements in an accurate and repeatable manner, the control elements and switching process have been analyzed to identify possibilities for improvement:

The Slide Button turned out to be a good control element with both high success and satisfaction rate. In contrast, the success rate of the Head Gesture was significantly lower, resulting in lower user acceptance. Furthermore, motion limitations negatively affect a user's ability to perform the Head Gesture correctly. The entire switching process was perceived as easy but slow, leaving room for improvement. As the Head Gesture has been perceived as difficult and has been in particular challenging for user's with restricted ROM, it should be discarded or improved in the future.

4. The HRI has to give sufficient and useful feedback to the user to allow safe and efficient operation.

The results of the study indicate that the calibration procedures are easy to understand and that sufficient and useful feedback is provided. The GUI was generally experienced as visually appealing and clearly structured. Moreover, the subjects agreed that all important functions could be accessed easily and all important information was displayed. A possibility to turn the sound off would be appreciated by most long-term users, though. In some cases, assessing the gripper position along the

^{w}z-axis was perceived as difficult. However, our experience indicates that users will learn to interpret the gripper camera image better after working with AMiCUS for a longer period of time. In conlusion, AMiCUS gives overall sufficient and useful feedback to the user to allow safe and efficient operation.

5. The HRI must enable the user to perform smooth, precise and efficient robot movements in Cartesian space.

Overall, the transfer function was well-adapted to most users during linear motion, rotation and gripping as it enabled accurate positioning while providing a suitable speed of operation. Therefore, AMiCUS enables the user to perform smooth, precise and efficient robot movements. In case the default settings are not suitable, the parameters of the transfer function can be adapted easily to meet the preferences of the user, in particular regarding operation speed.

6. The user should enjoy using the HRI.

User acceptance is often a critical point for assistive devices, jeopardizing their success as a product. AMiCUS, in contrast, received high user acceptance since the subjects of this study considered robot control with AMiCUS as fun.

In summary, AMiCUS fulfills all the requirements of a head-controlled HRI for robot arm control and has been greatly accepted by the subjects.

5.2. Comparison with Previously Published Work

When using the interface presented here, the user has to perform a Head Gesture and then activate a Slide Button in order to switch between robot groups. Even though the switching process can still be improved, switching will inherently take longer than for the interface presented by Jackowski et al. [29], which uses each one out of four different gestures to switch between robot groups. This direct group access makes switching very quick. However, the correspondence between gestures and robot groups depends on the current robot group, which is a general source of confusion and sometimes makes users select the wrong group. Furthermore, performing head gestures is complex and involves many muscles, some of which might not be available for tetraplegics with severe head motion limitations. As a matter of fact, out of 13 randomly picked tetraplegics, only 6 were capable to use the gesture-based interface presented by Jackowski et al. This strongly limits the applicability of this interface for individuals with head motion restrictions. Even more, if the restrictions are such that one or two head DOFs cannot be used for control: The interface presented within this work offers the possibility to change the mapping as described previously. This is hardly possible for the interface presented in Reference [29] because each new group resulting from a lost head DOF requires a new head gesture, whereas the ability to produce head gestures decreases with increasing head motion restrictions. For these reasons, we conclude that the interface presented by Jackowski is promising as a hands-free interface for people without head motion limitations, whereas the interface presented here is more suitable for individuals with head motion restrictions because it can be adapted to their special needs.

Supplementary Materials: The following are available online at http://www.mdpi.com/1424-8220/19/12/2836/s1, Static Data S1: 5 min of static data recorded with Hillcrest FSM-9, Dynamic Data S1: Head motion data recorded with Hillcrest FSM-9.

Author Contributions: Conceptualization, N.R. and M.G.; Data curation, N.R.; Formal analysis, N.R.; Funding acquisition, N.R. and M.G.; Investigation, N.R. and M.G.; Methodology, N.R.; Project administration, N.R. and M.G.; Resources, M.G.; Software, N.R.; Supervision, M.G.; Validation, M.G.; Visualization, N.R.; Writing—original draft, N.R.; Writing—review & editing, M.G.

Funding: This research was funded by the Federal Ministry of Education and Research of Germany grant number 01158324.

Acknowledgments: The authors would like to thank all the people involved, in particular Roland Thietje and his team from the BG-Hospital Hamburg, Axel Gräser, Icons8 and all the subjects who took part in the experiments.

Conflicts of Interest: The authors declare no conflict of interest.

Abbreviations

The following abbreviations are used in this manuscript:

AHRS	Attitude Heading Reference System
AMiCUS	Adaptive Head Motion Control for User–friendly Support
DOF	Degree of Freedom
GUI	Graphical User Interface
HMI	Human–Machine Interface
HRI	Human–Robot Interface
MEMS	Micro Electro-Mechanical System
ROM	Range of Motion
TCP	Tool–Center Point

References

1. Kirshblum, S.C.; Burns, S.P.; Biering-Sorensen, F.; Donovan, W.; Graves, D.E.; Jha, A.; Johansen, M.; Jones, L.; Krassioukov, A.; Mulcahey, M.; et al. International Standards for Neurological Classification of Spinal Cord Injury (Revised 2011). *J. Spinal Cord Med.* **2011**, *34*, 535–546. [CrossRef] [PubMed]
2. McDonald, J.W.; Sadowsky, C. Spinal-Cord Injury. *Lancet* **2002**, *359*, 417–425. [CrossRef]
3. Wyndaele, M.; Wyndaele, J.J. Incidence, Prevalence and Epidemiology of Spinal Cord Injury: What Learns a Worldwide Literature Survey? *Spinal Cord* **2006**, *44*, 523–529. [CrossRef]
4. Alsharif, S. Gaze-Based Control of Robot Arm in Three-Dimensional Space. Ph.D. Thesis, University of Bremen, Bremen, Germany, 2018.
5. Raya, R.; Rocon, E.; Ceres, R.; Pajaro, M. A Mobile Robot Controlled by an Adaptive Inertial Interface for Children with Physical and Cognitive Disorders. In Proceedings of the 2012 IEEE International Conference on Technologies for Practical Robot Applications (TePRA), Woburn, MA, USA, 23–24 April 2012; pp. 151–156. [CrossRef]
6. Lontis, E.R.; Struijk, L.N.S.A. Alternative Design of Inductive Pointing Device for Oral Interface for Computers and Wheelchairs. In Proceedings of the 2012 Annual International Conference of the IEEE Engineering in Medicine and Biology Society, San Diego, CA, USA, 28 August–1 September 2012; pp. 3328–3331. [CrossRef]
7. Rourke, M.; Clough, R.; Brackett, P. Method and Means of Voice Control of a Computer, Including Its Mouse and Keyboard. U.S. Patent 6,668,244, 23 December 2003.
8. Origin Instruments Corporation. Sip/Puff Switch User Guide. 2019. Available online: http://www.orin.com/access/docs/SipPuffSwitchUserGuide.pdf (accessed on 16 May 2019).
9. Graimann, B.; Allison, B.; Mandel, C.; Lüth, T.; Valbuena, D.; Gräser, A. Non-invasive Brain-Computer Interfaces for Semi-autonomous Assistive Devices. In *Robust Intelligent Systems*; Springer: London, UK, 2008; pp. 113–138.
10. Moon, I.; Lee, M.; Chu, J.; Mun, M. Wearable EMG-Based HCI for Electric-Powered Wheelchair Users with Motor Disabilities. In Proceedings of the 2005 IEEE International Conference on Robotics and Automation, Barcelona, Spain, 18–22 April 2005; pp. 2649–2654. [CrossRef]
11. Huang, C.N.; Chen, C.H.; Chung, H.Y. Application of Facial Electromyography in Computer Mouse Access for People with Disabilities. *Disabil. Rehabil.* **2006**, *28*, 231–237. [CrossRef]
12. Rupp, R.; Schmalfuß, L.; Tuga, M.; Kogut, A.; Hewitt, M.; Meincke, J.; Duttenhöfer, W.; Eck, U.; Mikut, R.; Reischl, M.; et al. TELMYOS—A Telemetric Wheelchair Control Interface Based on the Bilateral Recording of Myoelectric Signals from Ear Muscles. In Proceedings of the Technically Assisted Rehabilitation Conference (TAR 2015), Berlin, Germany, 12–13 March 2015.
13. Prentke Romich International, Ltd. Operator's Manual for the HeadMasterPlus. 1995. Available online: http://file.prentrom.com/122/HeadMaster-Plus-Manual.pdf (accessed on 16 May 2019).
14. La Cascia, M.; Sclaroff, S.; Athitsos, V. Fast, Reliable Head Tracking Under Varying Illumination: An Approach Based on Registration of Texture-mapped 3D Models. *IEEE Trans. Pattern Anal. Mach. Intell.* **2000**, *22*, 322–336. [CrossRef]

15. BJ Adaptaciones. BJOY Chin. 2019. Available online: http://support.bjliveat.com/en/productos/bj-853-en/ (accessed on 16 May 2019).
16. Raya, R.; Roa, J.; Rocon, E.; Ceres, R.; Pons, J. Wearable Inertial Mouse for Children with Physical and Cognitive Impairments. *Sens. Actuators A Phys.* **2010**, *162*, 248–259. [CrossRef]
17. Bureau, M.; Azkoitia, J.; Ezmendi, G.; Manterola, I.; Zabaleta, H.; Perez, M.; Medina, J. Non-invasive, Wireless and Universal Interface for the Control of Peripheral Devices by Means of Head Movements. In Proceedings of the IEEE 10th International Conference on Rehabilitation Robotics (ICORR), Noordwijk, The Netherlands, 12–15 June 2007; pp. 124–131.
18. Chen, Y.L. Application of Tilt Sensors in Human-Computer Mouse Interface for People with Disabilities. *IEEE Trans. Neural Syst. Rehabil. Eng.* **2001**, *9*, 289–294. [CrossRef] [PubMed]
19. Quha oy. Quha Zono Gyroscopic Mouse. 2019. Available online: http://www.quha.com/products-2/zono/ (accessed on 16 May 2019).
20. Music, J.; Cecic, M.; Bonkovic, M. Testing Inertial Sensor Performance as Hands-Free Human-Computer Interface. *WSEAS Trans. Comput.* **2009**, *8*, 715–724.
21. Mandel, C.; Röfer, T.; Frese, U. Applying a 3DOF Orientation Tracker as a Human–Robot Interface for Autonomous Wheelchairs. In Proceedings of the IEEE 10th International Conference on Rehabilitation Robotics (ICORR 2007), Noordwijk, The Netherlands, 12–15 June 2007; pp. 52–59. doi:10.1109/ICORR.2007.4428406. [CrossRef]
22. Williams, M.R.; Kirsch, R.F. Evaluation of Head Orientation and Neck Muscle EMG Signals as Three-dimensional Command Sources. *J. Neuroeng. Rehabil.* **2015**, *12*, 25. [CrossRef] [PubMed]
23. Fall, C.; Turgeon, P.; Campeau-Lecours, A.; Maheu, V.; Boukadoum, M.; Roy, S.; Massicotte, D.; Gosselin, C.; Gosselin, B. Intuitive Wireless Control of a Robotic Arm for People Living with an Upper Body Disability. In Proceedings of the 2015 37th Annual International Conference of the IEEE Engineering in Medicine and Biology Society (EMBC), Milan, Italy, 25–29 August 2015; pp. 4399–4402.
24. Kinova Inc.. KINOVA JACO—Assistive Robotic Arm. 2019. Available online: https://www.kinovarobotics.com/en/products/assistive-technologies/kinova-jaco-assistive-robotic-arm (accessed on 16 May 2019).
25. Rudigkeit, N.; Gebhard, M.; Gräser, A. Evaluation of Control Modes for Head Motion-Based Control with Motion Sensors. In Proceedings of the 2015 IEEE International Symposium on Medical Measurements and Applications (MeMeA 2015), Torino, Italy, 7–9 May 2015. [CrossRef]
26. Rudigkeit, N.; Gebhard, M.; Gräser, A. Towards a User-Friendly AHRS-Based Human-Machine Interface for a Semi-Autonomous Robot. In Proceedings of the 2014 IEEE/RSJ International Conference on Intelligent Robots and Systems (IROS2014), Chicago, IL, USA, 14–18 September 2014.
27. Rudigkeit, N.; Gebhard, M.; Gräser, A. A Novel Interface for Intuitive Control of Assistive Robots Based on Inertial Measurement Units. In *Ambient Assisted Living: 8. AAL Kongress 2015, Frankfurt/M, April 29–30, 2015*; Wichert, R., Klausing, H., Eds.; Springer International Publishing: Frankfurt/Main, Germany, 2016; pp. 137–146. [CrossRef]
28. Rudigkeit, N.; Gebhard, M.; Gräser, A. An Analytical Approach for Head Gesture Recognition with Motion Sensors. In Proceedings of the 2015 Ninth International Conference on Sensing Technology (ICST), Auckland, New Zealand, 8–10 December 2015. [CrossRef]
29. Jackowski, A.; Gebhard, M.; Thietje, R. Head Motion and Head Gesture-Based Robot Control: A Usability Study. *IEEE Trans. Neural Syst. Rehabil. Eng.* **2018**, *26*, 161–170. [CrossRef] [PubMed]
30. Zhang, L. Investigation of Coupling Patterns of the Cervical Spine. Master's Thesis, University of Dundee, Dundee, UK, 2014.
31. Hillcrest Laboratories, Inc. FSM-9 Modules, 2019. Available online: https://www.hillcrestlabs.com/products/fsm-9 (accessed on 16 May 2019).
32. The Qt Company. Qt | Cross-Platform Software Development for Embedded & Desktop. 2019. Available online: https://www.qt.io/ (accessed on 16 May 2019).
33. Universal Robots A/S. UR 5 Technical Specifications. 2016. Available online: http://www.universal-robots.com/media/50588/ur5_en.pdf (accessed on 16 May 2019).
34. Robotiq Inc. Robotiq 2F-85 & 2F-140 for CB-Series Universal Robots—Instruction Manual. 2019. https://assets.robotiq.com/website-assets/support_documents/document/2F-85_2F-140_Instruction_Manual_CB-Series_PDF_20190329.pdf (accessed on 16 May 2019).

35. Logitech Inc. Webcam C930e Data Sheet. 2017. Available online: http://www.logitech.com/assets/64665/c930edatasheet.ENG.pdf (accessed on 16 May 2019).
36. Wikipedia Contributors. Student's t-Test—Wikipedia, The Free Encyclopedia. 2019. Available online: https://en.wikipedia.org/w/index.php?title=Student%27s_t-test&oldid=898465472 (accessed on 16 May 2019).
37. Du Prel, J.B.; Röhrig, B.; Hommel, G.; Blettner, M. Choosing Statistical Tests: Part 12 of a Series on Evaluation of Scientific Publications. *Deutsch. Ärztebl. Int.* **2010**, *107*, 343–348. [CrossRef]
38. Wikipedia Contributors. Friedman Test—Wikipedia, The Free Encyclopedia. 2019. Available online: https://en.wikipedia.org/w/index.php?title=Friedman_test&oldid=890448021 (accessed on 16 May 2019).
39. Wikipedia Contributors. Fisher's Exact Test—Wikipedia, The Free Encyclopedia. 2019. Available online: https://en.wikipedia.org/w/index.php?title=Fisher%27s_exact_test&oldid=891629270 (accessed on 16 May 2019).
40. Wikipedia Contributors. Mann-Whitney U Test—Wikipedia, The Free Encyclopedia. 2019. Available online: https://en.wikipedia.org/w/index.php?title=Mann%E2%80%93Whitney_U_test&oldid=899337823 (accessed on 16 May 2019).

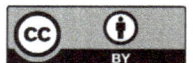

© 2019 by the authors. Licensee MDPI, Basel, Switzerland. This article is an open access article distributed under the terms and conditions of the Creative Commons Attribution (CC BY) license (http://creativecommons.org/licenses/by/4.0/).

MDPI
St. Alban-Anlage 66
4052 Basel
Switzerland
Tel. +41 61 683 77 34
Fax +41 61 302 89 18
www.mdpi.com

Sensors Editorial Office
E-mail: sensors@mdpi.com
www.mdpi.com/journal/sensors

www.ingramcontent.com/pod-product-compliance
Lightning Source LLC
LaVergne TN
LVHW070621100526
838202LV00012B/698